The
Disease Manager's
Handbook

Rufus Howe, RN, MN

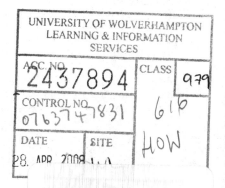

JONES AND BARTLETT PUBLISHERS
Sudbury, Massachusetts
BOSTON   TORONTO   LONDON   SINGAPORE

World Headquarters
Jones and Bartlett Publishers
40 Tall Pine Drive
Sudbury, MA 01776
978-443-5000
info@jbpub.com
www.jbpub.com

Jones and Bartlett Publishers Canada
2406 Nikanna Road
Mississauga, ON L5C 2W6
CANADA

Jones and Bartlett Publishers International
Barb House, Barb Mews
London W6 7PA
UK

Library of Congress Cataloging-in-Publication Data

Howe, Rufus S.
 The disease manager's handbook / Rufus Howe.
        p. ; cm.
Includes bibliographical references and index.
   ISBN 0-7637-4783-1
   1. Disease management–Handbooks, manuals, etc.   2. Outcome assessment (Medical care)
Handbooks, manuals, etc.   3. Patient education–Handbooks, manuals, etc.   4. Health
behavior–Handbooks, manuals, etc.
   [DNLM: 1. Disease Management–Handbooks.   2. Patient Education–Handbooks.
W 49 H857d 2005]   I. Title.
   RA394.H69 2005
    362.1–dc22   2004006395

Production Credits
Acquisitions Editor: Kevin Sullivan
Production Manager: Amy Rose
Associate Production Editor: Renée Sekerak
Editorial Assistant: Amy Sibley
Marketing Manager: Ed McKenna
Manufacturing and Inventory Coordinator: Amy Bacus
Composition: ATLIS Graphics
Cover Design: Kristin E. Ohlin
Printing and Binding: Malloy Inc.
Cover Printing: Malloy Inc.
Cover Image: © Photodisc

Printed in the United States of America
08 07 06 05 04   10 9 8 7 6 5 4 3 2

*To my wife Ruth
and our sons Christopher Paul and Gregory Scott*

Table of Contents

Foreword

> The future is literally in our hands to mold as we like. But we cannot wait until tomorrow. Tomorrow is now.
>
> *Eleanor Roosevelt*

DISEASE MANAGEMENT: THE EMERGING PROFESSION

Rarely are there individuals who see the future, can convey that vision to others, and can also plant and nurture the concepts that will develop through a profession. The author has crystallized here for each of us the outline for the present and provided a blueprint for the future for the professional disease manager. We are most fortunate to have such a clear-headed and complete outline of disease management practice within the vision of growth and development of disease management as a profession in such a succinct package!

There are those who might see disease management (DM) and case management (CM) as competing strategies. Far from that concept, our view is that the two strategies are complementary. As health care management efficiencies advance and cost-containment pressures continue to ramp up, DM and CM strategies may even be blended into an advanced and integrated model; yet before we can begin to understand the integration, each element of service delivery must be fully developed.

A clear need exists to begin the process of creating a professional structure for disease managers to include certification and a source for DM practice professional development.

> Disease Management is largely a business; but disease managers, who are the service delivery arm of that business, represent an emerging profession.
>
> *Rufus Howe*

DM AND CM: SIMILAR BUT DIFFERENT

Some similarities and many differences exist in the evolution of DM and CM professionals. Each professional group must put together the following elements—but not necessarily in this order—to enter into a professional status:

- Identification of a unique body of knowledge and the use of scientific methods to enlarge the body of knowledge
- Validation of a value proposition business case to positively contribute to improved clinical and financial outcomes—to deliver service and prove value to society
- Recognition and integration into the health care system
- Control of professional policy and professional activity
- Certification of individuals
- Accreditation of organizations
- Formalization of academic and continuing educational programs
- Formalization of standards of practice
- Development of an ethical code and industry-wide addressing of legal and ethical issues unique to the profession
- Industry research and continual improvement

While case management moved from practical application to science (we interact, we change behavior, we ask why and how to improve performance, and we gain technological support to enable research), disease management is moving into health care from science to application (we look at research, we seek to change behavior based on that research, and we interact).

CM looks at individuals within groups; DM looks at populations one person at a time. CM grew to a great extent through individual practitioners and was adopted by large organizations later supported by technical systems. DM has grown from large entities with technical-systems support to embrace and employ individual practitioners.

How Do We Relate?

In the whole of care management strategies, the two strategies are unique and complementary with shared common areas of practice in behavior change and care coordination skill sets. Disease management requires skills, academic and continuing educational support, and certification to distinguish it to the public as qualified at a level of practice.

The most effective way for that support to come together is through a professional society as this book so articulately outlines. A professional society provides a place of identity, where colleagues can share ideas, successes, identify emerging trends, tackle challenges with unity, and organize to move the profession forward.

As executive directors of the Case Management Society of America and the Disease Management Association of America, we welcome and respect disease managers as fellow professional colleagues. We pledge to you our support as you develop and grow. There is much case managers and disease managers share; there are also a number of differences. We will celebrate the blending of the two strategies and work together to make a difference in health care delivery.

We believe you will find this book of great value and a ready reference as you begin, or continue, your personal professional journey in disease management.

Jeanne Boling, MSN, CRRN, CDMS, CCM
Executive Director, Case Management Society of America

Warren E. Todd, MBA
Executive Director, Disease Management Association of America

Preface

At this moment there is a disease manager looking at his or her list of people to call or contact. They may be speaking to someone about doctor's instructions, encouraging their client to remember to take their medications on time or assuring a patient that their life will be filled with hope and expectation despite recent setbacks. The disease manager is not unlike the majority of health workers—filled with a desire to service their patients with expert knowledge, skills, and compassion.

What a rare privilege it is to be in a position to improve the lives of others. For me, this book represents a culmination of experiences that all point toward a similar passion to provide care and to do it for more than one person at a time. Starting with my first disease management program in 1983, I have always had the inclination to provide care to groups of people. At first, the groups were face-to-face and in relatively small numbers. Gradually, the number grew to 100, then to 1,000, and today, I am working for a company that actively manages over 1 million persons across the United States.

My first disease management program was designed for diabetics. I was a newly trained nurse practitioner practicing in an internal medicine clinic. My practice was filled with diabetics. I am told that in my first year I cared for over 6,500 of them! One thing was clear; my days were filled with redundancy. The diabetics had the same general pattern: multiple lifestyle and chronic condition issues that were laced with misunderstanding and confusion, with a healthy dose of self-defeating behaviors. It wasn't long before I realized that I was saying and doing the same thing from one 15-minute appointment to the next. What would happen if I said it once? Enter my first disease management program.

The diabetes program featured a full morning of instruction and discussion from a group of people—an ophthalmologist, dietician, podiatrist, dietician, and myself. We were a team that was hard to beat, and the patients loved it.

They were together, heard each other's questions, and were in the presence of a care team who provided expert counsel. This group met on a monthly basis to review treatment goals, learn a little more about diabetes, and even review their recent lab work and refill their prescriptions.

The popularity of this program caused us to hold multiple classes per week. The care team was caring for many more patients than was thought possible. The system in which we practiced required us to record the number and type of patients we saw each day. Once the program began, our individual statistics tripled, access to regular clinic visits improved dramatically, and of course, overall satisfaction with care was at an all-time high. This early diabetes program was rudimentary by today's standards, but it cemented in me the notion that disease management was a powerfully effective and efficient intervention.

My subsequent programs grew in size and sophistication. In 1986, I designed a cholesterol reduction program that was based on a recent National Institutes of Health clinical treatment algorithm. This program was instantly successful. The admonition to "Know Your Level" and the newly published Framingham study caused an obsession to understand one's cardiac risk. The Framingham study examined the rate of heart disease and its risk factors in a large group of people in Framingham, Massachusetts. One month after the flyer was posted in the hospital, over 3,000 patients signed up. The initial plan was to hold classes of 35 people—mostly driven by the number of chairs we had in our classroom. That wasn't going to work! We made design changes to include *calling* patients, larger classes, drop-in clinics, and graduation. Because of the intensity of this program, I decided to track the program on a personal computer using a simple database I had written especially for this purpose. This database grew into a network of health risk appraisal, lab, pharmacy, clinic visit, and clinical outcomes system that was used by all the hospital staff. Even though this program was a raging success with patients, there were big mistakes in the design of the program.

I found that, unlike the diabetes program, these patients didn't want to talk about their cholesterol long. Once they knew their cholesterol level and were on the road to reducing it, they had other issues that were not necessarily related to cholesterol. They weren't "cholesterol patients"; they were people with an elevated cholesterol level. It dawned on me that disease management was about people and not conditions. The condition is a mere portal of entry—a way to begin. What happens next is anyone's guess. That is easy to say, but in practice hard to design.

The next programs resulted in an evolution of design that attempted to accommodate all aspects of patient-centric design. Also, the various aspects of disease management that we know today became more formalized in my mind. Targeting, predicting, and identifying appropriate patients, separating patients into risk groups (stratification), creating smarter assessments, devising logic for care planning, understanding care giving approaches, and measuring the value of disease management have been my passion over the years.

The purpose for this book is to write it down for disease managers. My contention is that disease management is largely a business, but disease managers, who are the service delivery arm of that business, represent an emerging profession whose time has come. Disease managers will hopefully benefit from the thoughts and words in this book. Through this book and other related activities, perhaps we can begin the process of creating a professional structure for disease managers to include certification and a source for disease manager practice professional development.

Rufus Howe

About the Author

Rufus Howe has a background as an educator, exercise counselor, and internal medicine and family nurse practitioner. In these capacities, he has run a human performance laboratory, provided primary care, and participated in case and disease management initiatives. Howe has published texts and articles in a wide range of topics including clinical medicine, health promotion, health systems integration, case management, disease management, and clinical information system design. He has degrees from the State University of New York at Cortland (education), the University of Southern Maine (nursing), and the Oregon Health Sciences University (nurse practitioner).

Howe lives in Brentwood, Tennessee, with his wife Ruth and has two grown sons Christopher and Gregory. Rufus Howe is the vice president of product development for American Healthways, Inc., in Nashville, Tennessee.

Introduction

The disease management industry is growing by leaps and bounds. By some estimates, there are at least 3,500 persons in the United States who are working on the front lines of a disease management company, health insurance plan, or employer. Given the current growth trajectory of the disease management industry, this number may climb to more than 10,000 by the year 2010! In spite of the rapid growth of this area, little activity is occurring in the academic preparation, ongoing professional support, and certification for disease managers.

This growth is occurring at a time when the health care industry as a whole continues to struggle with structure and intent. Health insurance plans have become the largest purchasers of disease management services, largely driven by an increasing expectation from employers that the premium dollar will deliver more value than discounted services and traditional case management. According to carefully crafted outcomes models, the financial and clinical outcomes are largely positive.

One of the prime players in this equation is a person who is expected to deliver disease management interventions. Most of the time, this person has a basis in health care. They may be a nurse, pharmacist, dietician, social worker, health educator, or exercise physiologist to name a few possibilities. In this context, they are disease managers. Most persons in this role have had a full career fulfilling their root training, but have not had ample exposure to the knowledge and skills necessary to perform disease management. Given the complexity of delivering disease management services, there is ample room to further the distinct practice of disease management. This will require the formulation of a body of knowledge (beginning with this handbook), professional certification and recognition, and professional growth through continuing education, publications, and meetings.

The Disease Manager's Handbook serves at least two purposes. First, the handbook can be used as a textbook for prospective and current disease managers for training purposes. Each chapter contains learning objectives and challenge questions. When used in academic settings, the handbook can be used across a variety of courses or for one course. Further, no distinction or preference is made to a given profession, so nurses, pharmacists, and the like should derive equal value.

Second, the handbook sets the stage for the formalization of the disease management profession as a whole. There are emerging disease manager certification efforts underway as of this writing, and this handbook will be helpful to support those efforts.

Disease Management as a Business

For the most part, disease management is a business. Disease managers are the agents within this business that deliver the service. The business side is fairly well articulated throughout the industry.

The Disease Management Association of America (DMAA; www.dmaa.org) is an example of a prominent disease management organization, and describes itself in this way:

> The Disease Management Association of America is a non-profit, voluntary membership organization, founded in March of 1999, which represents all aspects of the disease management community.
>
> Creation of the association was in response to the continued growth of disease management in the United States. The increasing number of stakeholders dependent on the "promise" of disease management for cost effective, quality healthcare in the next millennium has created a need for a single voice and a more scientific approach to the measurement of the success of disease management programs.
>
> The mission of the Disease Management Association of America is to: "Advance Disease Management through standardization of definitions, program components and outcome measures; promote high quality standards for disease management programs, support services and materials; and educate consumers, payers, providers, accreditation bodies, and legislators on the importance of Disease Management in the enhancement of individual and population-based health."

The DMAA is mainly focused on industry issues, program design, and supporting the value of disease management. All of these are worthy and necessary goals, but fall short in promoting the actual practice of a disease manager. The DMAA is largely a trade organization.

Disease Management as a Practice

Disease management practice requires skills not unlike any other professional practice. Here is an example of how the state of Alabama describes nursing practice:

The performance, for compensation, of any act in the care and counseling of persons or in the promotion and maintenance of health and prevention of illness and injury based upon the nursing process which includes systematic data gathering, assessment, appropriate nursing judgment and evaluation of human responses to actual or potential health problems through such services as case finding, health teaching, health counseling; provision of care supportive to or restorative of life and well-being; and executing medical regimens including administering medications and treatments prescribed by a licensed or otherwise legally authorized physician or dentist. A nursing regimen shall be consistent with and shall not vary any existing medical regimen. Additional acts requiring appropriate education and training designed to maintain access to a level of health care for the consumer may be performed under emergency or other conditions which are recognized by the nursing and medical professions as proper to be performed by a registered nurse.

Using this Alabama example as a template, let's see what a disease management professional practice might look like in a similar professional regulatory context. The differences in the two examples are highlighted in boldface:

The performance, for compensation, of any act in the **predefined** counseling of **identified populations** in the promotion and maintenance of health and prevention of illness and injury based upon the **best-known medical evidence** which includes systematic data gathering, assessment, appropriate **clinical** judgment and evaluation of human responses to actual or potential health problems through such services as case finding, health teaching, health counseling; **coordination** of the provision of care supportive to or restorative of life and well-being; and **supporting** medical regimens including administering medications and treatments prescribed by a licensed or otherwise legally authorized physician or dentist. A **disease management** regimen shall be consistent with and shall not vary from any existing medical regimen. [Last sentence omitted.]

The differences between usual nursing and disease management practice should be obvious when these two descriptions are compared. This handbook provides disease managers a reference for their practice.

Like any profession, disease management has its own taxonomy and principles. The following question and answer section will help to clarify underlying principles used in this book.

Common Questions

- What is disease management?
  Disease management is a method used to apply best health care practices to a population—one person at a time. The goals of any disease management program are twofold:
  - To improve the health status of the patient

- To eliminate unnecessary medical utilization

  The impact of disease management is measured in terms of financial, clinical, and quality of life.

- Who pays for disease management?

  Health insurance companies, hospitals, clinics, pharmaceutical companies, and increasingly, the federal government, all count themselves as disease management sponsors.

- Who practices disease management?

  The disease management industry has a legion of practitioners on the phones, in clinics, on hospital floors, in pharmacies, in homes, and on the World Wide Web. Common names for these practitioners include disease manager, care manager, and population care manager. They are nurses, pharmacists, dieticians, social workers, health counselors, exercise physiologists, and respiratory therapists, to name a few.

- Is there a body of knowledge—apart from the usual training of these practitioners—that is required to engage in disease management practice?

  Yes. Disease management practice requires additional skills in finance, business, population targeting, sales, customer service, behavior change, social learning theory, educational strategies, marketing, and motivational interviewing.

- What is the professional preparation for disease managers?

  There is none. The current approach is either to train from within the sponsored organization or learn on the job. For many, it is the latter.

- Is there a professional organization dedicated to disease managers?

  No, not yet.

- Is there certification for disease managers?

  Yes, for pharmacists only. The certification, called a Disease State Management Certification, is administered through the National Institute for Standards for Pharmacist Credentialing. They can be contacted at the National Institute for Standards in Pharmacist Credentialling, 205 Daingerfield Road, Alexandria, VA 22314; 703-299-8790. Their Web site is www.nispcnet.org.

- When did disease management start?

  The truth is no one really knows when disease management started. There are many instances through history where a person or group instituted a health care program for the good of many. Certainly the early nursing pioneers and preventive health professionals were important early adopters. In post-modern times, disease management as we know it, took root in the mid-1990s. It is probably better to say that disease management is here and here to stay.

Terms

Like any profession, the disease management profession has its own lingo. Because the meanings of words are sometimes confusing, let's go through the more common terms used in this book. Each term will be defined and clarified. A deeper look into concepts surrounding each will be provided throughout the book.

Care planning. Care planning is the act of producing the care plan. Disease managers may do this through predefined rules using guidelines or algorithms. Professional judgment may also play a central role in the care-planning process. Of special note, goal writing is part of care planning.

Caregiving. Caregiving is the tangible evidence of care planning. The disease manager has multiple methods of caregiving. These include telephone counseling, mailed materials, and health team interaction.

Clinical information system (CIS). The clinical information system is the software that disease managers use to track and record their work. Not all disease managers use or need a CIS do their work, but they are in the minority.

Disease manager. The term "disease manager" is used throughout the book. This role is well described in the literature and has wide acceptance in the industry. Is there a better name for this profession? Perhaps. The main problem with the name is that as the science and application of disease management matures, the concept of managing a disease is giving way to managing a person. Another common objection to this name is that it doesn't sound right for a disease manager to work in a maternity, health promotion, or prevention program. Rarely do two words perfectly describe such a profession, and disease manager is a good example of that. Therefore, for the purpose of clear and consistent communication, disease manager is the name of the profession for this book—warts and all.

Economic modeling. Economic modeling is the process by which the disease manager determines if a program makes sense economically. Income and expenses are compared to ensure the viability of the program.

Fulfillment. Fulfillment is mailed materials. Workbooks, educational material, and letters are all fulfillment. In the near future, fulfillment will extend to e-mail and reading material that is placed on a secure web site.

Person (people). "Person" is used to denote the object of all disease management programs. Some settings like to use "member" because that is what a health plan calls its customers; others prefer "patient" or "client." Disease managers speak to a person about their clinical situation. They may be a member of a health plan, a client of a case manager, and a patient of their physician. We'll call them a person.

Population.   Population has many meanings, unfortunately. Used alone, population means the *entire* population under management of the sponsor. All persons in a health plan's commercial line of business constitute a population. On the other hand, a group of diabetics selected from the population becomes the targeted population.

Predictive modeling.   Predictive modeling is a mathematical process that quantifies a person's likely future health costs compared to others in the population. Predictive modeling is most often used as a population targeting strategy and is a form of segmentation. This science is evolving and is thought to have significant promise for disease management.

Return on investment (ROI).   The return-on-investment analysis measures the financial impact of the disease management programs. A ROI of 1:1 means that the impact of the program (return) equaled the program cost (investment). A ROI of 2:1 means that the impact of the program doubled the money invested in the program.

Segmentation.   Segmentation is the result of a rules-based grouping of people in a population. One might use rules to divide a population by cost, utilization parameters, or clinical patterns. Segmentation is frequently used to presort a population into more manageable groups.

Stratification.   Stratification is a dynamic assessment of a person's status. It is used for a variety of purposes such as determining contact frequency or care-planning elements. Persons are stratified through assessments, lab values, events, or other real-time inputs. Stratification is different from segmentation in that segmentation occurs automatically, at regular intervals, and with the same rules.

CHAPTER 1

Disease Management Context and Model

─────────── **OBJECTIVES** ───────────

After reading this chapter, the reader will be able to:
1. Describe the basic attributes of disease management practice.
2. Articulate the conceptual location of a disease manager within the whole of health care.
3. List the five major plans of care that a disease manager must coordinate and reconcile.

OVERVIEW

The purpose of this chapter is to lay out general principles for the context of disease management and propose a conceptual model of where disease managers fit within the whole of health care.

Disease management, as defined in this handbook, is conceptually located outside the point of care. If this is true, then it is clear that disease managers do not engage in prescriptive activity, do not physically treat or care for a person, and are not considered a primary care provider in any definition of that term. Disease managers are the ultimate observers, advocates, and coordinators of care.

One can say that disease management practice has attributes that are common to all forms of disease management. The primary attributes are:

- **Approach** to the person is rooted and heavily affected by the context of the disease manager's initial professional training.
- **Interventions** are based upon known science—sometimes known as evidence-based medicine. When there is no agreed-upon best practice, follow the best opinion from thought leaders in the field. Whatever the

1

source of knowledge, the clinical content is considered the official recommendation.

- **Interactions** are with a population who have similar characteristics such as condition, age, gender, health status, financial utilization, or health risk. This attribute implies proactive, preventive interventions.
- **Communications** are structured to a predefined outline of instruction or rule sets based upon the targeted population.
- **Behavior change** is a primary outcome of disease management practice. The object of change is not limited to the person, but also includes health care team members, facilities, risk-bearing organizations, and governmental agencies.
- There are **predefined clinical outcomes** that are central to the value of the initiative. Increasing the medication adherence rate for a population with hypertension is one example.
- **Relationships** with other health care providers or facilities do not require formalization. No requirement exists for all parties to depend on each other. The disease manager resides at the hub of the care coordination wheel.
- **Longitudinal interactions** are driven by health status or by a set of predefined parameters.

DISEASE MANAGER APPROACH

Disease managers approach their practice in many ways. Pharmacists, for instance, are trained to interact in a way that differs from social workers. This is appropriate because of the context of the interaction and the probable subject matter of the discussion. A pharmacist is unlikely to do a family support evaluation or a social worker to discuss potential drug interactions.

The core of the approach lies in the initial professional training of the disease manager. The refined approach is a function of the disease management setting. There are instances where the approach does not require any substantive alterations—such as nurses performing blood pressure checks in a health fair. There are, however, times when the approach may differ significantly. One common setting is seen in the telephonic disease management used by disease management vendors. Typically, the approach requires acquisition of new skills such as cold calling, selling techniques, and motivational interviewing to name a few.

INTERVENTION SOURCES

Interventions come from the best science possible. For the most part, this means evidence-based medicine (EBM). This is not an issue for the common disease-managed conditions such as diabetes and chronic obstructive pulmonary disease. It becomes an issue for other lesser-understood conditions such as fibromyalgia.

Dr. David Sackett, founder of Canada's first department of clinical epidemiology at McMaster University, states that EBM is "the conscientious, explicit, and judicious use of current best evidence in making decisions about the care of the individual patient. It means integrating individual clinical expertise with the best available external clinical evidence from systematic research."[1]

Disease managers use EBM to guide decisions meant to provide appropriate care. Even though the origins of EBM are in medical literature, the application of this knowledge must be compared to clinical reasoning, individual circumstances, and personal choices.

EBM continues the work of the research that produced it. Put another way, disease managers are a manifestation of EBM. The intervention is performed in the context of three variables: (1) clinical expertise, (2) patient values, and (3) the best evidence. Most EBM is a result of experimental trials. Simply put, this means the researchers used accepted methodologies that prove beyond chance that the intervention should work.

Important features of the strongest research designs include ensuring that ethical considerations are in place, the research question builds upon prior validated knowledge, the study population is appropriate in composition and size, the comparison groups are as similar as possible, the groups are assigned in a random fashion, the intervention and measurement is reliable (consistently measures the same event) and is valid (uniquely measures the attribute in question), the statistical tests are appropriate for the study data, and finally, the results are described considering potential limitations to the study itself.

TARGET POPULATION

One primary assumption of disease management is that the population shares a characteristic. The population doesn't have to be limited to a condition. The main reason for this requirement is to focus on the proposed objective of the disease management program; for instance, increasing the rate of measles immunizations requires an age requirement.

COMMUNICATION

What and when to communicate are functions of the disease management design, with the disease manager as the agent of that design. Once the target population is identified, the design consists of inputs (clinical assessment, utilization data, lab values, etc.), throughputs (rules that test for patterns of data), and outputs (care plans, interaction intensity). This structure ensures consistent application of best practices across a population. Mass customization is the most appropriate way to think of this attribute.

KNOWLEDGE AND SKILL TRANSLATION

Disease managers are asked to translate rather complex medical knowledge into digestible and actionable items for persons in their care. This is not an easy task. The common vehicles for this activity are verbal instruction, written educational materials, and perhaps video. Like any communication, there is a sender and a receiver. The constant is that the sender conveys reliable and valid content. The variable is whether the recipient understands and internalizes the content.

The usual mechanism to ensure effective translation is the return demonstration of knowledge. Examples of this include if the person can state the four symptoms of a heart attack, describe how to reverse a hypoglycemic reaction, or state why exercise is important to a diabetic. Knowledge transfer is but one small piece of the equation. Knowledge does not reliably lead to behavior or positive clinical outcomes, but knowledge is foundational to sustained behavior change.

BEHAVIOR CHANGE

Influencing health-promoting behavior is, by far, the most difficult aspect confronting the disease manager. Behavior change science is weak despite the wealth of applied research. Tobacco use has generally reduced over the years due to many factors, some of which are directly attributable to behavior change interventions. Obesity, however, is rampant. It is a significant challenge to motivate an obese person to reduce calories and become more active.

Disease managers are at the forefront of behavior change. The future behavior change research will focus on the various interventions disease managers use. This will mean that a key attribute of a disease manager will be their ability to influence behavior change.

OUTCOMES

"Begin with the outcome in mind" is the mantra for disease manager designers and the guiding principle for disease managers. Outcomes can be thought of as either process or end point outcomes. Process outcomes are milestones within the process that lead to a final result. An example of a process outcome is the rate of hemoglobin a1c testing in a population. In this context, the blood test is part of an assessment process upon which the primary provider makes treatment decisions and the person gauges their progress toward diabetic control.

An end point outcome is the final result. An example of an end point outcome is the rate of strokes in a population of persons with atrial fibrillation. In this case, the rate of strokes is a result of interventions that have altered the measurement. Be careful to choose end point outcomes that are truly end points. For example, the rate of patients taking anticoagulants is more likely a process outcome because it has a direct effect on the rate of strokes.

RELATIONSHIPS TO HEALTH CARE TEAM

One interesting attribute of a disease manager's practice is where they are in relationship to other entities who affect the person. In the case of disease managers who fit into the common chronic aspect of practice, there are at least five major entities: the physician, the person, the medical evidence, the regulatory agencies, and the risk-bearing agencies. All of these entities have their own plan of care and rarely do these plans match. Table 1.1 and Figure 1.1 illustrate how each plan of care may play out for a person with high blood cholesterol and coronary artery disease.

Once viewed in this light, it is obvious that the disease manager's role is to bring the various plans of care into a workable solution that benefits the person as well as the other entities. Because the disease manager's efforts focus on the person's orientation, this task is particularly difficult. The average person has no idea what the other plans of care do or should contain. The disease manager, in this context, is required to keep all this in mind during the process.

LONGITUDINAL CARE

Disease managers are likely to have more than one interaction with a person over time. The program design may have preset intervals (call every 14 days), predefined lessons or steps, or open access to persons engaged in the program. The longitudinal nature of disease management practice calls for a sense of progression that is hopefully positive and orderly. Most disease management programs measure progress with a series of milestones such as reassessments, repeated data capture, or a series of outcome measures.

One important factor in disease management practice is the meaning of actively engaged. Most disease management programs have clear entry points that are driven by identification parameters. Some programs have clearly defined exit or gradation criteria that are driven by measurable end point outcomes such as not smoking for 6 months. Chronic illness programs have a harder point to define. Most programs assume that despite best efforts,

Table 1.1 The Disease Manager's Relationship to the Health Care Team

Orientation	Plan of Care	Comments
Self-care	Eliminate potato chips; walk stairs, not take elevator at work; try and beat problem without having to take medications for the rest of their life.	Personal strategies are powerful in their likelihood of success, but may be self-defeating or limited in scope.
Primary care	Draw lipid sample; check blood pressure; give Lipitor 20mg at bedtime; return to the clinic in 3 months to retest lipids; stop smoking.	Tough to conduct exhaustive evaluation and provide adequate education in a 15-minute office visit.
Medical evidence (condensed for illustration purposes)	Trial of step 1 low fat diet for 3 months; assess LDL target-based on-risk profile; assess for and educate on risk-factor reduction; assess for evidence of active coronary artery disease; consider angiogram; check thyroid status; check blood pressure, treat with BP over 120/70 with combination of lifestyle and medication; avoid tobacco; limit alcohol; regular exercise.	All items are relevant to this person. If followed, will significantly decrease their morbidity, and perhaps prevent premature death.

Table 1.1   The Disease Manager's Relationship to the Health Care Team (*continued*)

Regulatory agency (National Committee for Quality Assurance, Utilization Review Accreditation Commission, Joint Commission on Accreditation of Healthcare Organizations)	Provide mechanism for goal setting; track progress toward goals; provide screening recommendations (HEDIS).	Calls for processes that are difficult for point-of-care settings and are challenging for risk-bearing agencies.
Risk-bearing agency	Prefer generic medications over name brand; assess higher cost to upper tier medications; yearly physicals not covered; must meet criteria before conducting angiogram; smoking cessation aids may not be covered in benefits; cardiac rehabilitation visits up to 3 months post MI, no more than 20 visits.	Earnestly desires a lower aggregate risk for its insured population. Benefit structure may positively or negatively impact best practices. One size does not fit all situations, and existing systems are inadequate to tailor benefits to individual circumstances.

Figure 1.1   The Disease Manager's Relationship to the Health Care Team

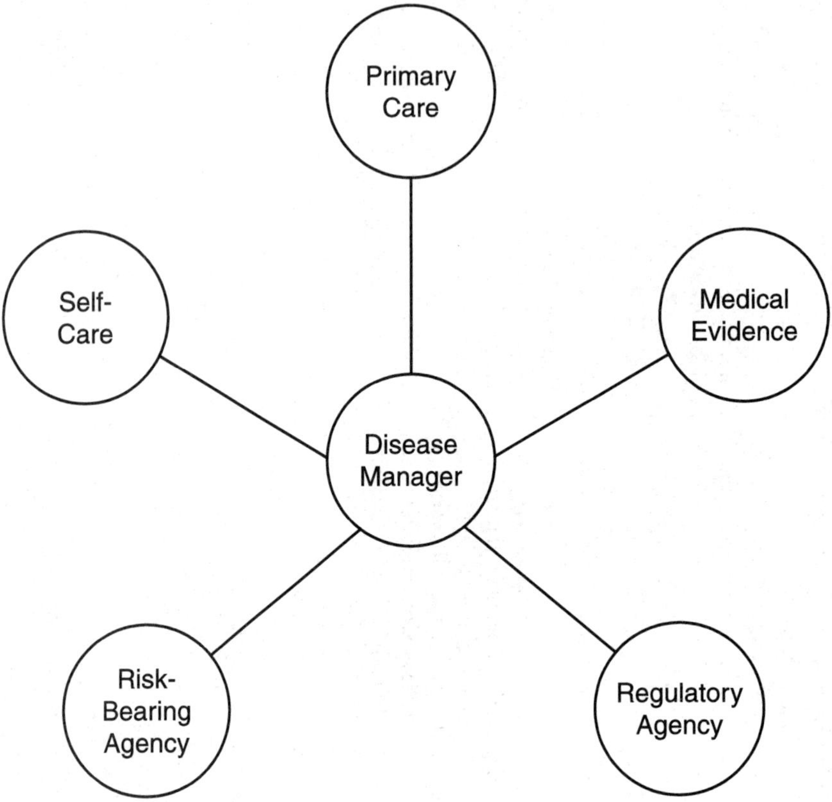

the illness will have greater functional impact as time wears on and member-ship in the program will continue until death or other forced exit reasons.

Obviously, the role of a disease manager is critical and requires substantial knowledge of where they fit within the whole. No matter what the initial train-ing of the disease manager or the setting for disease management, the factors outlined in this chapter have relevance for all situations. As the industry and practice matures, the understanding of how these factors come together in an optimal way will emerge.

The next steps for the disease management professional evolution are to ensure that programs have designs that lead to measurable interventions, are conducive to accurate data capture, and provide feedback mechanisms for future improvements. This will require disease managers who are trained and have the inclination to conduct research in the area of their practice.

Like any model, this one will have to stand the test of time and professional scrutiny. The objective is to begin the discussion, then refine as the understanding grows.

CHALLENGE QUESTIONS

1. To what degree can a disease manager impact the day-to-day behavior of a physician they will never meet?
2. To what degree are disease managers prepared to influence behavior change? Are there reliable tools or interventions to support disease managers?
3. How well does the health care system as a whole monitor a person with chronic illness?
4. Why is there a need for a disease manager?
5. Is evidence-based medicine a realistic foundation for disease management practice?

Endnotes
1. Sackett, D. *Evidence-Based Medicine: How to Practice and Teach EBM*, 2nd ed. London: Churchill Livingstone, 2000.

CHAPTER 2

The Past, Present, and Future of Disease Management

———— **OBJECTIVES** ————

1. Briefly describe key events that have affected disease management to the present day.
2. List several predicted future events in disease management and for disease managers.

OVERVIEW

When the notion of disease management actually was introduced is up for some debate. One can argue that if you consider attempts to care for a population of ill persons, then it is possible to trace this kind of activity back to the earliest times. Public health initiatives have attempted to influence the health status of a population for as long as public health has been around. In her 1863 *Notes on Hospitals*, Florence Nightingale, a nursing pioneer, recognized and advocated for efforts to bring a population's health into better control.[1]

This chapter could be extremely long and involved. There were and are many twists that have affected disease management over the years. Relevant events and points are presented to give the disease manager a feel for their legacy and provide a basis upon which to move to the future.

DISEASE MANAGEMENT PAST

This chapter will start with the contemporary understanding of disease management and will begin at a rather inauspicious place: health statistics and health statisticians. In the early 1960s, a physician named Kerr White published a paper on "The Ecology of Medical Care."[2] In this paper, Dr. White demon-

11

strated that there were predictable utilization patterns among those in the at-risk population. In summary, the results showed that for every 1,000 adults from the at-risk population, about 750 of them will report an illness or injury during a 1-month period, 250 will see a physician, 9 will be admitted to a hospital, and 1 will be referred to a university medical center. The distribution of this population has not changed since this first study.

This data compelled health systems to determine the reasons for this troubling phenomenon and to attempt to put mechanisms in place to improve the situation. Two subsequent events catapulted disease management into the forefront. First, pharmacy companies realized that there were huge opportunities to ensure persons with chronic illness were taking their medications at the right doses and for the right length of time, and secondly, managed care organizations started to bear risk for populations causing them to have a financial interest in their members' health status.

Pharmaceutical companies were the first to offer large scale disease management programs. These programs were usually offered at no to low cost and were designed around appropriate drug treatment. Lifestyle issues were addressed, but did not dominate the approach. Early on, these programs were mail based and touted huge numbers of persons who received the mailings. Later, a few of these companies experimented with telephonic disease management with minimal success.

The advent of the managed care boom in the mid-1980s to mid-1990s coupled with spiraling health care costs spawned new interest in refining the health care insurance industry. Because of strict regulations, these companies could not limit their insured population to healthy persons, so actuaries developed health premium pricing schemes that would in effect use the healthy member's premium dollars to fund the cost of the ill or injured members. This arrangement worked, but as time went by, the cost of health care per member rose faster than expected and essentially broke the actuarial assumptions.

Because this trend had the potential to bankrupt the health plans, other avenues of reducing health costs had to be put in place. The earliest initiatives included case management and utilization management. Case management, in this context, focused on care coordination of the sickest health plan members in an attempt to reduce unnecessary costs while preserving the overall quality of care. Utilization management was another initiative that used predetermined clinical criteria to approve or decline specific procedural or hospitalizations when requested.

Pharmacy-based disease management programs sprung up in the early 1990s. Health plans began to build their own disease management programs with people from their case management departments shortly thereafter. By

1996, several disease management companies started to offer their services. The early conditions targeted by these companies were diabetes, asthma, and heart failure. Hospitals, feeling the trend to perform more outpatient surgeries and noticing declining revenues overall, also began disease management programs in hopes of offering extra services that would route patients back to the hospital.

Disease managers in this era were pioneers; there were no precedents. Quite often, disease managers were the designers, developers, and clinicians all rolled into one. The disease management practice consisted of examining new assessments, new interventions, and new contact frequencies. Incredibly, the disease management industry grew from a random and uncoordinated effort to a practice that today is cohesive and standard throughout the industry.

Despite the hard and excellent work, there was a pall growing over disease management in the form of value. For too many reasons to list, the first disease management efforts were not able to present savings data with confidence. Internal and external initiatives came and went over the inability to demonstrate savings. The commercial disease management companies recognized this as a true threat to their business and set forth to prove its value. The concerted effort of financial, data, and clinical experts silenced the naysayer with solid data that did in fact prove that the presence of disease management in a population positively impacts clinical and financial data.

DISEASE MANAGEMENT PRESENT

Today, disease management is in evidence across a wide variety of settings and conditions. Advances in technology and data handling have significantly improved the ability to provide disease management to a huge number of persons. Although the data is almost impossible to validate, recent estimates are that there almost 2 million lives under active management in the United States.

Disease managers have made good use of remote home monitoring, home visit services, Web interfaces, and telemonitoring. It is not unusual to see a disease manager check on the blood pressure and weight of a patient many miles away, call them if a value is out of bounds, and get them back on track.

Disease management training has also improved greatly. The industry has gone from little or no training to full-fledged training sessions, sometimes lasting up to a month. Pharmacists have established training and certification, and there are university-based efforts to do the same with nurses and other allied health providers.

DISEASE MANAGEMENT FUTURE

The future direction of disease management will depend on at least three areas: (1) technology advances, (2) the professionalism of the disease manager, and (3) program savings models.

The future disease management systems will incorporate deep analytical risk tools that consider financial and clinical data in order to stratify patients into urgency groups. The clinical information systems will rival the personalization engines of Amazon.com. In this way, every patient will be treated as unique. Remote patient monitoring will extend to smart cell phones, PDAs, and even home checkup stations. The use of secured Web and e-mail will proliferate.

The emerging profession of a disease manager will gain a foothold. This book is one evidence of this trend; there will be more like it in the future. Colleges and universities will offer disease management programs of study. Professional organizations will cater to disease managers rather than disease management. National competency-based disease manager certifications will also be available.

Program savings models will challenge current program designs. There will be significant shifts in contact rates, intensity of interventions, and more efficient program platforms. The disease management sponsors (primarily health plans and large employers) will force research that will measure disease management as an intervention and expose still more opportunity to impact a population.

CHALLENGE QUESTIONS

1. Do you agree that disease management is about to dramatically increase its depth and breadth?
2. Will new technology threaten disease manager positions?
3. If managed care as we know it goes away, what will happen to disease management?

Endnotes

1. Nightingale, F. *Notes on Hospitals*, 3rd ed. London: Longman, Green, & Roberts, 1863.
2. White, K., Williams, T., and Greenberg, G. The ecology of medical care. *New England Journal of Medicine* (1961). 265:885–92.

Disease Management Program Designs

OVERVIEW

When the more recent influx of disease management programs came on the scene, there was one design: Form a list of people who have the same disease and have the appropriate health professional speak with them. Fortunately for the industry, designs have evolved to match the value proposition at hand.

Today, these program designs are much more elegant and are still improving. The improved designs are a function of differing program objectives, settings, resources, and funding. The most popular design categories are high acuity, common chronic, other chronic, rare chronic, screening, and primary prevention.

Disease managers can find themselves working within many different approaches. The approach may be guided by any or all of the value propositions. Table 3.1 describes how the approach affects the value proposition.

HIGH ACUITY DISEASE MANAGEMENT

The high acuity model typically focuses on the top 1 to 3 percent of the high cost population. The interventions are based on avoiding events such as hospitalization, emergency room use, or high cost procedures. The patients are identified proactively through specialized identification algorithms that

Table 3.1   Disease Management Approach and Value Proposition

	Examples	Financial	Clinical	Education	Satisfaction
High Acuity	High cost patients; high predictive model scores.	Hospital and emergency department cost avoidance.	Coordination of care; intense communication between the entire team.	Short bursts of key learnings to satisfy the present situation.	Entire team's perception is important.
Common Chronic	Diabetes; heart failure; COPD; coronary artery disease; asthma; ESRD.	Total medical expenditures reduced through best practice care.	Rates and values of key clinical tests; symptom and functional improvement.	General self-management skills; specific monitoring skills; risk reduction.	Patient emphasized; physician data is a bonus.
Other Chronic	Low back pain; hepatitis C; atrial; fibrillation; osteoporosis.	Same as chronic. May segment costs based on condition.	Symptom control; functional status.	Background knowledge and skills related to the condition.	Patient is emphasized.
Rare Chronic	Myasthenia gravis; Rheumatoid arthritis; cystic fibrosis; ALS, etc.	Costs related to medications, procedures, certain hospitalizations.	Symptom control; functional status; lab metrics.	Specific monitoring and self-management skills.	Patient and physician; possibly other team members.

Table 3.1   Disease Management Approach and Value Proposition (*continued*)

Screening	Hepatitis C; depression; diabetes; cancer; mammogram; bone densitometry.	Total medical expenditure across 3- to 5-year time horizon.	Positive screening rate; condition stage when found.	Awareness of condition; risk avoidance measures.	Patient and employer.
Health Populations	Knowledge acquisition; symptom triage; health coaching.	Total medical expenditure across 3- to 5-year time horizon; focus on redirection of utilization.	Service utilization.	General education; episodic and situation dependant in nature.	Patient and employer.
Primary Prevention	Seat belt use; tobacco; preconception; folic acid.	Utilization costs of specific events related to primary prevention topic.	Avoidance of adverse clinical events specific to primary prevention topic.	Specific to primary prevention topic.	Patient and employer.
Pharmaceutical	Polypharmacy; complex medication.	Adherence rate per identified medication.	Rate of adverse reactions per identified medication.	Education specific to medication.	Patient.

may or not have a predictive component. The main difference between this disease management approach and others is that it is not condition based.

High acuity disease management is the closest thing to case management of all the models thus far. Patients are as sick and are as complex but the main difference is that, unlike case management, these patients were identified proactively. Nurse disease managers have almost no difficulty moving to this model because it most closely matches their training and nursing practice.

High acuity patients do not stay long on the disease manager's list. They die, move to another segment of the care management process, or get better. Case list or registry management is paramount in this model. A patient must stay on the case list for only as long as required to create the value (cost avoidance). This is sometimes a difficult thing to do because of the unpredictability of what the near term future might hold for a patient with this degree of medical complexity. In this model, creating value is at its peak for a short time. Value in this sense is created when the disease manager's interventions are effectively improving health status, reducing unnecessary utilization, or improving the quality of life for the patient.

Disease managers will have a one-to-one relationship with their patients and may even be assigned to a physician group for ease of operation.

COMMON CHRONIC DISEASE MANAGEMENT

Common chronic disease management targets patients with diabetes, heart failure, coronary artery disease, chronic obstructive pulmonary disease, or end stage renal disease. This form of disease management is characterized by high volume identification, education, and support services. The disease manager's primary role is to ensure the best practices are followed within the condition category.

Disease managers in this model work for health plans or disease management vendors and are thus in the high volume business. The notion is to connect with as many patients as possible to maximize the value propositions. Connecting with many patients is both a challenge and a costly proposition. Industry rates for connectivity hover around 30 percent for the commercial population and somewhat higher for the older Medicare population.

For this reason, predictive modeling, segmentation, and stratification form the basis for how these patients are operationally managed. The seasoned disease management program becomes quite adept at presorting, sorting, and sorting again its patients before a disease manager makes a connection. Clearly, the skill in common chronic disease management is to speak to the right person at the right time, then say the right thing!

Common chronic disease management is relatively straightforward for disease managers. Each condition has a set of key clinical indicators, knowledge, and behaviors to learn. A clinical information system captures the data by means of automated assessments and perhaps care plans that appear based upon preordained rules.

Because this model relies heavily on heightening the awareness and facilitating behavior change for patients who require further intervention, disease managers are required to be motivational interviewers, coaches, and some would say, salespersons.

There may be as many as 25 disease managers working on a team that covers 5,000 to 8,000 patients. This may not seem very patient friendly, but the model works well when the information system can pick up where the last disease manager left off, creating continuity between the two interactions.

OTHER CHRONIC DISEASE MANAGEMENT

A relatively new trend exists that applies common chronic disease management methodologies to other diseases. The other chronic conditions may include acid-related stomach disorders (dyspepsia, peptic ulcer disease, gastritis), atrial fibrillation, decubitus ulcer, hepatitis C, inflammatory bowel disease, irritable bowel syndrome, osteoporosis, osteoarthritis, and urinary incontinence.

These additional conditions have imparted an interesting aspect to the more traditional close cousin, the common chronics. This aspect has more to do with the patient's situation than the condition itself.

RARE CHRONIC DISEASE MANAGEMENT

Rare chronic disease management usually includes conditions such as seizure disorders, rheumatoid arthritis, multiple sclerosis, parkinson's disease, systemic lupus erythematosus, myasthenia gravis, sickle cell anemia, cystic fibrosis, hemophilia, scleroderma, polymyositis, chronic inflammatory demyelinating polyneuropathy (CIDP), amyotrophic lateral sclerosis, dermatomyositis, and Gaucher disease.

The underlying premise is that although these conditions are rare, they are devastating to the person and costly to the health care system. For this group of conditions, gaps in care mirror the common chronic model even though these persons are followed by highly trained subspecialists. In all cases, there are opportunities to readdress and refine treatment options, improve self-management, and increase health care team support. In some cases, network or pharmaceutical benefit design may play a role in improving care.

Rare chronic disease managers are asked to have a deep knowledge of each of the conditions they manage. It is entirely possible that disease managers in this model subspecialize for instance, only handling patients with Gaucher disease. Due to the nature of these conditions, physician and pharmacist integration is critical to the success of this model. Disease managers work either in small teams or have a primary relationship with the person. This design is also likely to have the most varied disease manager team composition—registered nurses, dieticians, pharmacists, social workers, and so forth.

SCREENING

Screening disease management programs typically include depression, immunizations, mammogram, cancer, heart disease, and hepatitis C. Disease managers rarely participate in screening activities as a primary focus of their duties, but this design bears mentioning because the tide is slowly turning in this direction. The primary issues with screening programs are the relatively longer return on investment and difficulty in connecting with enough people to make a difference.

The mechanisms for screening usually do not involve a verbal connection between the disease manager and the screening population. Instead, paper surveys, interactive surveys, or voice-response technologies are used. The results of these screenings are then provided to the person and the agency that did the screening. The disease manager then becomes more of a health coach using informed decision-making techniques to counsel the person on what to do about their positive screening result.

PRIMARY PREVENTION

Like screening programs, disease managers rarely engage in primary prevention programs. Examples of a primary prevention program include seat belt use, fire alarms, radon detectors, and birth control. Also like screening programs, the cost and return on investment of these programs is not conducive to the usual disease management sponsor groups.

PHARMACEUTICAL

Pharmacists practice disease management in a variety of ways. On a population level, they monitor medication trends, correcting gaps in prescribing, and also minimizing potential abuses in medication use. Pharmacists work with disease management programs to ensure appropriate medication therapy is in place on a case-by-case basis. One can argue that each time a pharmacist hands a prescription to a person and provides education about that medication, they are performing as a disease manager.

CHALLENGE QUESTIONS

1. How do disease managers utilize the skills of social workers?
2. What is the difference between a case manager and a disease manager?

CHAPTER 4

Value Proposition for Disease Management

 OBJECTIVES
---

1. Define what is meant by value proposition.
2. List the major areas to consider when constructing a return on investment model.
3. Describe how disease management settings affect measuring disease management effectiveness.
4. Explain, in simple terms, regression to the mean.

OVERVIEW

Simply stated, a value proposition is a statement of proposed worth. Relating to disease management, a program's value proposition may be to reduce total medical expenditures through reducing hospital visits. The value proposition reflects the work necessary to meet the stated goal. The following equations provide examples of how this works using a disease management example in ever-increasing granularity:

Disease management interventions = Reduced hospitalizations

Population targeting + just-in-time interaction + focused interventions
= Reduced hospitalizations

Predictive modeling + daily authorization data + tailored plans of care
= Reduced hospitalizations

For the most part, value propositions are based upon scientific evidence of past value. For instance, if there is data that supports a similar intervention causing a reduction in hospitalizations, then there is high confidence in this value proposition. However, because disease management is relatively new in its modern form, there are still value propositions that have a lower confidence level. A value proposition that calls for increased employee creativity may be true if measured, but there is little evidence that it is true if it is not measured. Thus a lower confidence level is anticipated.

The value proposition for disease management has at least four major components: (1) clinical, (2) financial, (3) educational, and (4) satisfaction. New employer-centric trends in disease management are adding absenteeism, presenteeism, and productivity measures to the mix.

CLINICAL VALUE

Disease management delivers tremendous clinical value. Examples of tangible clinical value are improved lab measurements or a reduction in pain scores. Disease managers are in a unique position to influence clinical aspects of care. They are not physically at the point of care, yet are asked to ensure a particular lab test is done, for instance. Normally, one thinks of a clinical intervention as a hands-on, face-to-face activity. For the most part, the disease manager is not able to see their patient, limiting the power of a clinical interaction. The clinical value proposition is dependent on the ability of the disease manager to assess, plan, and move the patient and physician to do something clinically positive from a remote position. Strategies to accomplish this value are mentioned later in the book and are central to the disease manager practice.

FINANCIAL VALUE

Almost without exception, disease management provides financial value to the sponsor of the services. Typically, health risk-bearing organizations such as managed care organizations or self-insured companies sponsor disease management to help curb escalating health costs. The cost savings don't stop at the sponsor; very often the patients benefit as well through lower medication costs, fewer procedures, or reduced clinic visits. The premise is that both sides of the equation win when disease management is done correctly. Disease managers deliver the goods—they are the agent, the means to the end, and the cornerstone of the value creation.

EDUCATIONAL VALUE

Deriving an educational value proposition is an interesting proposition in itself. Certainly disease managers must spend time educating, and certainly education is important, but what is uncertain is the relationship between knowledge acquisition and the rest of the value equation. Knowing why one should monitor their blood glucose may or may not affect blood glucose monitoring behavior, for instance. Disease managers can measure differences in understanding using pre/post testing. The value of education must be taken into context. Education is a process step that may lead to better clinical, financial, and satisfaction scores.

SATISFACTION VALUE

Satisfaction is a value proposition that has multiple purposes. Most would agree that patients who are satisfied are more likely to trust their caregivers, have a positive outlook, and are loyal to their physician and health plan. The fact that the disease manager is an agent or advocate for the key stakeholders is not lost on the people who measure disease management programs. Happy patients lead to a stable business.

DISEASE MANAGEMENT VALUE PER PROGRAM DESIGN

Disease managers work in many settings. The sources of the value will differ by disease management program design. The program design and objectives will guide any or all of the value propositions. Table 4.1 describes how the design affects the source of the value proposition.

DETERMINING THE VALUE OF DISEASE MANAGEMENT

Now that the various aspects of a value proposition are understood, it is time to turn to how this value is designed into a program. Disease management designers use a model that incorporates a combination of factors that when tied together, demonstrate the value of the program. When a disease manager engages a person to educate, support, or motivate them, the work behind the value proposition is sometimes lost.

The following example provides insight on how these factors relate to each other and will be used for the remainder of the chapter. The scenario is based upon a request to formulate a disease management program for diabetic persons. In this example, there are registered nurses, dieticians, and a pharmacist on staff. The model is telephonic and the sponsor is a large employer.

Who Is in the Group?

The first task is to determine members of the group. Normally, the identification is from medical claims data and in this example that is true. The employer has a population of 100,000 persons (employees and their dependents),

Table 4.1   Sources of Disease Management Value Proposition per Approach

	Examples	Clinical	Financial	Education	Satisfaction
High Acuity	High-cost patients; high predictive model scores.	Coordination of care; intense communication between entire team.	Hospital and emergency department cost avoidance.	Short bursts of key learnings to satisfy present situation.	Entire team's perception important.
Common Chronic	Diabetes; heart failure; COPD; coronary artery disease; asthma; ESRD.	Rates and values of key clinical tests; symptom and functional improvement.	Total medical expenditures reduced through best practice care.	General self-management skills; specific monitoring skills; risk reduction.	Patient emphasized; physician data a bonus.
Other Chronic	Low back pain; hepatitis C; atrial fibrillation; osteoporosis.	Symptom control; functional status.	Same as chronic; may segment costs based on condition.	Background knowledge and skills related to the condition.	Patient emphasized.
Rare Chronic	Myasthenia Gravis; rheumatoid arthritis; cystic fibrosis; ALS.	Symptom control; functional status; lab metrics.	Costs related to medications, procedures; certain hospitalizations.	Specific monitoring and self-management skills.	Patient and physician; possibly other team members.

Table 4.1   Sources of Disease Management Value Proposition per Approach (*continued*)

Screening	Hepatitis C; depression; diabetes; cancer; mammogram; bone densitometry.	Positive screening rate; condition stage when found.	Total medical expenditure across 3- to 5-year time horizon.	Awareness of condition; risk avoidance measures.	Patient and employer.
Health Populations	Knowledge acquisition; symptom triage; health coaching.	Service utilization.	Total medical expenditure across 3- to 5-year time horizon; focus on redirection of utilization.	General education; episodic and situation dependant in nature.	Patient and employer.
Primary Prevention	Seat belt use; tobacco; preconception; folic acid.	Avoidance of adverse clinical events specific to primary prevention topic.	Utilization costs of specific events related to primary prevention topic.	Specific to primary prevention topic.	Patient and employer.
Pharmaceutical	Polypharmacy; complex medication.	Rate of adverse reactions per identified medication.	Adherence rate per identified medication.	Education specific to medication.	Patient.

and their ages range from newborn to 65 years old. Using national prevalence data for this group, we know that the prevalence is 6 percent or 6,000 out of 100,000 persons will likely have diabetes. We also know that a national average of total claims cost for diabetes is approximately $4,300 per year. Given these factors, we will estimate that the total cost burden for the employer is $25,800,000 for their diabetics. Generally speaking, cost estimates include all medical costs, not just those associated with the disease in question. This is due to the difficulty in reliably associating medical costs to a single condition; this brings the discussion to disease burden and the way disease management programs arrive at selecting the target population.

Epidemiologists have rather sophisticated models for estimating disease burden. Simply put, disease burden is the sum of the financial and clinical cost of a particular disease. This is usually expressed in terms of prevalence and direct and indirect costs.

Prevalence is the number of patients in a population that have the condition. Here is an example of prevalence: "Approximately 18.2 million people, 6.3 percent of the population, have diabetes." Disease management efforts usually start with finding the prevalence in the target population. This entails developing a set of search criteria (wrongly called an algorithm in the industry) against a medical claims database that may look something like this:

Header Information

    Ages: all ages

    Place of service: all places of service

    Number of hits: 2 hits in any 12-month window

    Position: any position

ICD-9 Codes: Any patient with any of the codes in Table 4.2. (Note: ICD-9 codes are a standard list.)

Data analysts use this information to search through all patient data to find people who fit these search criteria. Notice that this search criterion uses a two-hit rule. This means that a patient must have two claims for any of the ICD-9 codes mentioned in the search criteria in a 12-month time window.

Incidentally, disease managers bear the brunt of the accuracy of these data runs. The mark of excellent search criteria is few false positive and negative results. Disease managers do not want to be put in the position of mentioning a condition to a patient when they in fact do not have it. The limitation to this method is that a person can have two of these claims and not have the condition due to a medical workup that did not yield a diagnosis.

Once the data run is complete, the result is the target population prevalence. This number almost never matches the national numbers for many rea-

Table 4.2   ICD-9 Member Identification Codes

ICD-9 Code	Description
250	Diabetes mellitus -Excludes: gestational diabetes (648.8) hyperglycemia NOS (790.6) neonatal diabetes mellitus (775.1) nonclinical diabetes (790.2) that complicates pregnancy, childbirth, or the puerperium (648.0)
250.0	Diabetes mellitus without mention of complication Diabetes mellitus without mention of complication or manifestation classifiable to 250.1–250.9 Diabetes (mellitus) NOS
250.1	Diabetes with ketoacidosis Diabetic: acidosis without mention of coma ketosis without mention of coma
250.2	Diabetes with hyperosmolarity Hyperosmolar (nonketotic) coma
250.3	Diabetes with other coma Diabetic coma (with ketoacidosis) Diabetic hypoglycemic coma Insulin coma NOS -Excludes: diabetes with hyperosmolar coma (250.2)
250.4	Diabetes with renal manifestations Use additional code to identify manifestation, as: diabetic: nephropathy NOS (583.81) nephrosis (581.81) intercapillary glomerulosclerosis (581.81) Kimmelstiel-Wilson syndrome (581.81)
250.5	Diabetes with ophthalmic manifestations Use additional code to identify manifestation, as: diabetic: blindness (369.00-369.9) cataract (366.41) glaucoma (365.44) retinal edema (362.83) retinopathy (362.01–362.02)
250.6	Diabetes with neurological manifestations Use additional code to identify manifestation, as: diabetic: amyotrophy (358.1) mononeuropathy (354.0–355.9) neurogenic arthropathy (713.5) peripheral autonomic neuropathy (337.1) polyneuropathy (357.2)
250.7	Diabetes with peripheral circulatory disorders Use additional code to identify manifestation, as: diabetic: gangrene (785.4) peripheral angiopathy (443.81)

Table 4.2   ICD-9 Member Identification Codes (*continued*)

ICD-9 Code	Description
250.8	Diabetes with other specified manifestations Diabetic hypoglycemia Hypoglycemic shock Use additional code to identify manifestation, as: diabetic bone changes (731.8) Use additional E code to identify cause, if drug-induced -Excludes: intercurrent infections in diabetic patients
250.9	Diabetes with unspecified complication
251.0	Hypoglycemic coma Iatrogenic hyperinsulinism Non-diabetic insulin coma Use additional E code to identify cause, if drug-induced -Excludes: hypoglycemic coma in diabetes mellitus (250.3)
251.1	Other specified hypoglycemia Hyperinsulinism: NOS ectopic functional Hyperplasia of pancreatic islet beta cells NOS -Excludes: hypoglycemia in diabetes mellitus (250.8) hypoglycemia in infant of diabetic mother (775.0) hypoglycemic coma (251.0) neonatal hypoglycemia (775.6) Use additional E code to identify cause, if drug-induced
251.2	Hypoglycemia, unspecified. Hypoglycemia: NOS reactive spontaneous -Excludes: hypoglycemia with coma (251.0) in diabetes mellitus (250.8) leucine-induced (270.3)
253.5	Diabetes insipidus Vasopressin deficiency -Excludes: nephrogenic diabetes insipidus (588.1)
271	Disorders of carbohydrate transport and metabolism -Excludes: abnormality of secretion of glucagon (251.4) diabetes mellitus (250.0–250.9) hypoglycemia NOS (251.2) mucopolysaccharidosis (277.5)
271.4	Renal glycosuria Renal diabetes
275.0	Disorders of iron metabolism Bronzed diabetes Hemochromatosis Pigmentary cirrhosis (of liver) -Excludes: anemia: iron deficiency (280.0–280.9) sideroblastic (285.0)
276	Disorders of fluid, electrolyte, and acid-base balance -Excludes: diabetes insipidus (253.5) familial periodic paralysis (359.3)

Table 4.2   ICD-9 Member Identification Codes (*continued*)

ICD-9 Code	Description
337.1	Peripheral autonomic neuropathy in disorders classified elsewhere / Code also underlying disease, as: amyloidosis (277.3) diabetes (250.6)
357.2	Polyneuropathy in diabetes / Code also underlying disease (250.6)
358.1	Myasthenic syndromes in diseases classified elsewhere Amyotrophy from stated cause classified elsewhere Eaton-Lambert syndrome from stated cause classified elsewhere / Code also underlying disease, as: botulism (005.1) diabetes mellitus (250.6) hypothyroidism (244.0–244.9) malignant neoplasm (140.0–208.9) pernicious anemia (281.0) thyrotoxicosis (242.0–242.9)
362.0	Diabetic retinopathy / Code also diabetes (250.5)
366.41	Diabetic cataract / Code also diabetes (250.5)
443.81	Peripheral angiopathy in diseases classified elsewhere / Code also underlying disease, as: diabetes mellitus (250.7)
581.81	Nephrotic syndrome in diseases classified elsewhere / Code also underlying disease, as: amyloidosis (277.3) diabetes mellitus (250.4) malaria (084.9) polyarteritis (446.0) systemic lupus erythematosus (710.0) -Excludes: nephrosis in epidemic hemorrhagic fever (078.6)
583.81	Nephritis and nephropathy, not specified as acute or chronic, in diseases classified elsewhere / Code also underlying disease, as: amyloidosis (277.3) diabetes mellitus (250.4) gonococcal infection (098.19) Goodpasture's syndrome (446.21) systemic lupus erythematosus (710.0) tuberculosis (016.0) -Excludes: gouty nephropathy (274.10) syphilitic nephritis (095.4)
588.1	Nephrogenic diabetes insipidus -Excludes: diabetes insipidus NOS (253.5)
648.0	Diabetes mellitus [0-4] Conditions classifiable to 250 -Excludes: gestational diabetes (648.8)

Table 4.2   ICD-9 Member Identification Codes (*continued*)

ICD-9 Code	Description
648.8	Abnormal glucose tolerance [0-4] Conditions classifiable to 790.2 Gestational diabetes
731.8	Other bone involvement in diseases classified elsewhere / Code also underlying disease, as: diabetes mellitus (250.8)
751.7	Anomalies of pancreas Absence of pancreas Accessory pancreas Agenesis of pancreas Annular pancreas Ectopic pancreatic tissue Hypoplasia of pancreas Pancreatic heterotopia -Excludes: diabetes mellitus: congenital (250.0–250.9) neonatal (775.1) fibrocystic disease of pancreas (277.00–277.01)
775.0	Syndrome of "infant of a diabetic mother" Maternal diabetes mellitus affecting fetus or newborn (with hypoglycemia)
775.1	Neonatal diabetes mellitus Diabetes mellitus syndrome in newborn infant
775.6	Neonatal hypoglycemia -Excludes: infant of mother with diabetes mellitus (775.0)
785.4	Gangrene Gangrene: NOS spreading cutaneous Phagedena Use additional code for any associated condition, as: diabetes (250.7), Raynaud's syndrome (443.0) -Excludes: gangrene of certain sites– see Alphabetic Index gangrene with atherosclerosis of the extremities (440.24) gas gangrene (040.0)
V18.0	Diabetes mellitus
V65.3	Dietary surveillance and counseling Dietary surveillance and counseling (in): NOS colitis diabetes mellitus food allergies or intolerance gastritis hypercholesterolemia hypoglycemia obesity
V77.1	Diabetes mellitus

Source: International Classification of Diseases, Ninth Revision, Clinical Modification (ICD-9-CM), 2004. National Center for Health Statistics, 3311 Toledo Road, Hyattsville, MD 20782. (301) 458-4000. http://www.cdc.gov/nchs/icd9.htm

sons. For those who are not aware, office coding systems are not well controlled and physicians and their office staff may neglect to record the correct ICD-9 code.

It is clear that the employer spends quite a bit on diabetes every year. The next step is to determine if there are opportunities to improve the health of the diabetics enough to justify the cost of delivering the program. In fact, the opportunities are at the core of what a disease manager does.

What Are We Going to Improve?

There are gaps in care with every condition; diabetes is not alone in that regard. Program designers will perform extensive literature searches that describe the outstanding issues—or gaps in care—for diabetes. The literature search must be consistent with the primary aim of the program—to improve health status, thus decreasing unnecessary expenditures.

The opportunity section is the most inexact portion of the value equation. The issues that can go right or wrong with a person are endless. One can decide to ascribe a general number to this section and move on or attempt to identify and quantify the issues. The former approach would simply say that there is a problem with diabetic care, and this program will improve the situation by 20 percent. The latter approach—and the one this scenario will take—is what are the primary issues facing diabetics, and what kind of impact can be made in each of these areas?

Our example identifies four primary issues: heart attack, stroke, renal failure, and amputation. There are many other medical issues that diabetics face including obesity, arthritis, infection, depression, hypertension, and blindness to name a few. This example chooses to concentrate on the first four because they represent large impact areas and are areas in which a disease manager can have significant impact.

For each section, there is literature backing for the incidence rates (rate of new cases each year) and costs per event. Using the heart attack example, we see that 4 percent or 240 persons out of the 6,000 diabetics in the program will have a heart attack in the next year. Based on an average cost of $34,000 per heart attack event, this would equate to $8,160,000 per year. The program expects to reduce the cost of heart attacks by 10 percent a year. That equates to a cost savings of $816,000 per year for this population.

Disease managers will, as a central part of their program, remind their clients to stop smoking, lose weight, get regular exercise, take an aspirin a day, monitor their blood pressure and cholesterol, and know the signs of a heart attack. These are example interventions that are buried in the mind of the program designer when they arrive at the impact value.

The remainder of the opportunity section is formatted the same way and describes the issues and impacts per the other major issues. Based on the four opportunities, a potential exists to save $1,291,890. What is not accounted for are the ancillary benefits gained from disease manager interaction such as general health improvement that will lead to generally lower health utilization. The example does not account for this effect and is thus a conservative estimate of impact.

What Are We Going to Do?

Now that the opportunities are laid out, the program interventions start to take shape. The program designers will construct delivery options that are amenable to the target population. Notice, for instance, that there is a provision for home visits to a small portion of the population. This is because data analysis shows that a small segment of the diabetic population is home bound due to pressure ulcers or other debilitating conditions.

The program design calls for a combination of telephonic contact, mailing, and home visits. Each cost has its own attributes that will be somewhat unique to every setting. For purposes of this example, let us assume that, on average, a diabetic will receive three calls per year lasting 12 minutes each. Using a cost of $3.00 per minute to deliver such services, the calling cost of this program is $648,000. (For the curious, the $3.00 per minute includes all costs relating to staffing including salary, benefits, and all operational costs. This is a sobering calculation and is at the heart of why the disease manager's time is carefully managed.)

Mailing costs are straightforward. Each member will receive three mailings a year at a cost of $4.50 each, totaling $81,000. The mailing costs are small compared to the calling figure, but the relative impact may be as well.

The remaining cost is home visits. Only 1 percent of the population, 60 persons, will receive a visit. At a cost of $75.00 each, this will total $4,500.

Return on Investment

The example states a 1.76-to-1 return on investment. This represents the benefit of the program divided by the cost. In other words, the return on investment is like income: for every $1 invested, $1.76 is returned after 1 year. Not a bad investment and disease managers are in the middle of the intervention that will make this happen. To put things in context, most disease management programs have a 1.0- to 2.0-to-1 return on investment. Figure 4.1 shows how this looks when applied to a spreadsheet format.

Figure 4.1   Diabetes Value Proposition (Example Only)

Who is in the group?		
Total population	100,000	
Prevalence	6%	
Target diabetic population	6,000	
Average cost per year (total)	$ 4,300	
Total diabetes cost burden		**$ 25,800,000**
What are we going to improve?		
Heart attack rate		
Incidence	4%	
Number affected	240	
Cost per person	$ 34,000	
Total cost	$ 8,160,000	
Proposed impact	10%	
Cost after savings	$ 7,344,000	
Amount saved		**$ 816,000**
Stroke rate		
Incidence	2%	
Number affected	108	
Cost per person	$ 29,000	
Total cost	$ 3,132,000	
Proposed impact	12%	
Cost after savings	$ 2,756,160	
Amount saved		**$ 375,840**
Renal failure		
Incidence	0.25%	
Number affected	15	
Cost per person	$ 29,000	
Total cost	$ 435,000	
Proposed impact	15%	
Cost after savings	$ 369,750	
Amount saved		**$ 65,250**

Figure 4.1   Diabetes Value Proposition (Example Only) (*continued*)

Amputation				
Incidence		0.10%		
Number affected		6		
Cost per person	$	29,000		
Total cost	$	174,000		
Proposed impact		20%		
Cost after savings	$	139,200		
Amount saved			$	34,800
What are we going to do?				
Call				
Times per year		3		
Minutes per call		12		
Cost per minute	$	3.00		
Total calling charge			$	648,000
Mail				
Times per year		3		
Cost per person	$	4.50		
Total mailing charge			$	81,000
Home visit				
Persons requiring visits per year		1%		
Cost per visit	$	75.00		
Total mailing charge			$	4,500
Total savings			$	1,291,890
Cost of delivery				
Total charge for program			$	733,500
Overall savings			$	558,390
Return on investment				1.76:1

Regression to the Mean

If there is an albatross around the disease management industry's neck, it is regression to the mean. This is a phenomenon that the disease manager is almost too close to see first hand. A short explanation of regression to the mean will bear this out.

Regression to the mean is a statistical phenomenon that applies to populations who are nonrandom and the measurements have questionable reliability and validity. In disease management, this manifests itself when we target a chronically ill population (nonrandom) and attempt to measure the population using medical claims as a surrogate for better care (imperfect due to wide variation in the coding and data systems that produce medical claims).

Regression to the mean can be illustrated using a simple example from a high school physical education class. Let's say that we choose a group of high school students who are in the lowest 10 percent for times in the 1-mile run; their average running times are far below the average. Let us also say that our program to help them run faster is ineffective (we do nothing). If that is true, then the running times shouldn't change much. However, when measured again 6 months later, the group's average scores have indeed improved, they have moved—or regressed—to the mean!

How did this happen? First, the composition of the group will not be stable. Some students will leave the group through natural improvements, desire, and maturity, and some will enter the group through lessening skills. There is little chance that the same students will remain in the lowest running time group. Whatever the movement, the original group will always move toward the mean, giving the appearance of improvement where none actually is.

If the group was randomly selected, they would represent the typical or normal distribution of the larger population. Disease management interventions performed on this group would better demonstrate impact. If a group is selected based on the law of averages, that is right where they will stay. The mind-boggling aspect of regression to the mean is when you apply two measures to a nonrandomized group, which is almost always the case in disease management, the scores seem to always improve. The further the group is away from the mean, the larger the effect will be in either direction. This happens anytime there are two measures across time in a nonrandom population.

The last major factor affecting regression to the mean is the accuracy of the measure itself. In disease management, this includes medical claims, lab values, and other self-reported data. There is significant measurement error in all these categories, and thus Measurement 1 and Measurement 2 will not correlate well. The reasons behind this are somewhat complex and warrant more in-depth study.

Proving the Value Proposition

The value of disease management as stated earlier is the confluence of many factors and, as just described, complicated by others. Because of the inherent difficulty with applying highly rigorous experimental design to disease management, many programs have adopted using general, rather than specific, indicators for success. One example of this is a medical cost trend that entails calculating the trends of costs of a given population, then measuring the actual trend for the measurement period. The result of this calculation should be a difference in costs, called cost avoidance, or the money *not* spent on a group.

Another mechanism to proving value is to measure clinical values as rates in a pre/post fashion. For instance, tracking pre- and post-Hba1c values gives an indication of the effectiveness of an intervention to remind persons to get regular Hba1c tests.

Disease managers spend most of their time on the front line of the program, not behind the scenes crafting return on investment evaluations or program effectiveness results. Even though this is true, disease managers would greatly enhance their own effectiveness by understanding the basic principles of value creation and how value is measured along the way.

CHALLENGE QUESTIONS

1. What can a disease manager do to reduce the effect of regression to the mean?

2. What are the most important factors in the value proposition for disease managers to know when they are engaging clients?

3. Is there a way to capture most of the opportunities in the return on investment calculation, rather than focusing on a few major ones?

CHAPTER 5

Telephonic Disease Management

———————— OBJECTIVES ————————

1. List the major points of a telephonic interaction.
2. Describe ways to promote successful engagement.
3. Explain the purpose and techniques for assessment data collection.
4. Describe at least five assessment possibilities of medication intervention.
5. Explain the purpose and components of care planning and how they relate to caregiving.

OVERVIEW

A large percentage of all disease management is conducted over the phone. Disease managers, especially those who have spent their career working in direct care environments, find telephonic interactions to be challenging. The five senses are reduced to one, hearing, and that can be frustrating. This chapter outlines a basic approach to telephonic disease management call flow that can be applied to almost any program design.

ENGAGEMENT: THE FIRST CALL

By far the hardest part of telephonic disease management is the first call. Because disease management is supposed to be proactive—taking action before the event—the first call is generally not the idea or desire of the person on the other end of the phone. Often, the person may be hesitant to begin a relationship with a stranger around such a sensitive problem as health. The recent influx of telemarketing calls has not helped either. Many persons who answer the phone and do not know the caller are understandably skeptical about the intent of the service. In this manner, the term pro-active is certainly not always a well-received concept.

Resistance to help is a somewhat foreign concept for most health care providers who are in constant demand in other arenas. Hospital nurses are used to answering to call buttons; pharmacists are in great demand to give instruction about a medication; and dieticians regularly are held in high regard for their services. Therefore, the notion that a person will not want or trust a call from one of these professionals is a hard thing to grasp and causes a great deal of angst for disease managers.

Engagement then is a cross between selling and creating instant value for the person. The typical disease manager is not a salesperson, had sales training, or has the "thick" skin to deflect the natural tendency not to trust the caller. The following includes several techniques, borrowed from sales and engagement specialists, that are helpful to learn and master:

1. If you truly don't believe that you are a valuable agent for a service that will changes lives, you will struggle.
2. Be confident—sound confident.
3. Gender bias is in effect! A warm compassionate voice is interpreted differently by men and women. Learn to tailor your manner to the gender.
4. Do not read your introduction script! In fact, it is best to sound as casual as possible without appearing too friendly.
5. Identify yourself clearly and slowly as a registered nurse, dietician, or pharmacist and allow that to sink in. This is a powerful statement. Rarely do people *receive* calls from people with your training. You might introduce yourself as: "Hello, Mr. Jones. This is Martha Greene. I'm a registered nurse calling on behalf of Acme Health Plan."
6. Do not say anything further until the person acknowledges that they have heard you. Most will not say many words, but use the short silence to build curiosity about why you would be calling them.
7. Introduce the purpose of your call in plain language, and then wait for the response. "The purpose of my call is to let you know about a **free service** that is designed to provide health support to its members (patients, etc.)."
8. Because most disease management programs are sponsored by parent organizations, they are free. The person you are calling should know this up front. Also, try hard not to mention any identifying information at this time. If a person hears that you know they have diabetes, heart problems, or asthma, they will start wondering how you know this information and a distrust will build before you start. The fact is that most people with conditions would choose not to become a member of

a disease management service if they knew it was only for persons with a certain condition. They don't think of themselves as a diabetic, for instance. Most persons would, however, opt for a program that ensures they will be as healthy as possible.

9. Listen. Allow for the member to engage **you** in the conversation. They may mention something about the sponsoring agency, perhaps positive or even negative. Be assuring and actively listen. Most people cannot talk for more than 90 seconds without repeating themselves. If you listen at least 90 seconds, you create an illusion of a great listener and will gain early trust points.

10. Allow the person to reveal their medical information. Many people will open up and reveal an amazing amount of information without probing, especially those who have active disease.
    a. Sample response from a person: "You're a nurse from Acme Health Plan. Well, I'm surprised that they are doing this. I have had trouble getting answers about my last hospital bill. Anyway, what's going on with this program?"
    b. Another possibility: "I received a letter about this a week ago. Sounds like a good thing for people who need it—not sure I do. What is this all about?"
    c. Another possibility: "You are a nurse? My wife's a nurse as well. She makes sure that I take my pills every morning. I'm not sure I need another nurse! My wife is here to help with me things if I need it. What are you supposed to do?"

    There are innumerable responses, and they will range from the very positive to the very negative. In the end, it doesn't matter. The person is in early thinking mode about what you have said and doesn't really have a firm basis upon which to agree to continue.

11. Always assume that the person will cooperate to some degree with you.

12. If the person has not opened up to the health-related issue about which you are calling, start with some open-ended questions.
    a. "Mr. Jones, I am here to provide you with health information. What would you like to know about?"
    b. Or: "Mr. Jones, lots of people struggle to some degree with their health. I know that medical help can be confusing—what's on your mind?"

13. Keep the nature of the disease management program general. Try to cover broad topics such as education and support services, helping the patient think through health-related activities, and supporting the physician with helpful clarifications.

14. Do not talk a lot on the first call. Let the person believe that they will be the active participant.

15. The first call should be brief. Give the potential client enough information to satisfy their understanding of who you are and what might happen. If possible, introduce the subject of the next call in a way that will create interest in what they are about to experience.

16. Schedule a date and time window for your call. Ask the person to write it down where they are used to keeping track of future events.

17. Ensure basic demographic data.

18. Try to document one personal thing about the member that you learned. Perhaps you heard a dog barking and learned the dog's name, the person may have said they were about to visit their son in Iowa, and so forth. If you mention this to the person on the next call, they will feel you care about them enough to engage them on a personal level.

CLINICAL INFORMATION: THE SECOND CALL

The second call may require a little reselling, reconfirmation, and overall reminding. Once that is complete, the next step is to begin to understand the clinical picture of the person. This explanation assumes that the disease manager knows very little about the person except their basic demographic data and perhaps their identifying condition.

Current Status

"How are you doing today?" is a great starting question. If the answer is "Fine" or "I'm doing very well," then move on to the next section. If they say that they are having problems, it is worth guiding them through this process. An orderly collection of data will ensure future credibility. The "OLDCART" mnemonic is a tried and true way to collect meaningful clinical information. The following is an example exchange using this technique.

Disease Manager: How are you doing today?

Mr. Jones: My legs are starting to hurt.

Disease Manager: When did that start? (Onset)

Mr. Jones: About 3 weeks ago.

Disease Manager: Where on your legs does it hurt? (Location)

Mr. Jones: From my knees down—on both legs.

Disease Manager: Do they hurt all the time? (Duration)

Mr. Jones: Not at first, but they do now.

Disease Manager: How would you describe the pain? (Character)

Mr. Jones: My legs throb—sometimes they feel like I just hit them on a coffee table.

Disease Manager: Is there anything that makes the pain worse? (Aggravating factors)

Mr. Jones: When I sit for a long time and forget to raise my feet.

Disease Manager: Is there anything that makes the pain better? (Relieving factors)

Mr. Jones: Yes—when I have to walk a lot, the pain seems to subside a bit.

Disease Manager: Have you tried anything to get rid of this pain? (Treatments)

Mr. Jones: Only Advil but that doesn't seem to work.

Medications

Collecting medication information is extremely valuable but time consuming. Most experienced disease managers will tell you that this can often be the longest part of the phone call, especially for the older person. For this reason, the objective for collecting medication information should be carefully considered. Do not assume that a totally complete medication evaluation is necessary in all cases. Remember the context of disease management: It is outside the actual point of care.

In this area, disease managers—and those who design disease management programs—need to challenge themselves. We have probably gone overboard in our zeal to collect medication information for large segments of the population. It may be because disease managers are trained to be diligent in this area during their training and in their experience prior to participating in disease management. They may be carrying through with what they know; therefore, the habit continues. However, there is not a one-size-fits-all requirement in this area.

For instance, to what degree does the program depend on a correctly dosed person? If the bulk of the program's value position is to avoid hospitalization through early symptom identification, then knowing exact, real-time dosing is probably not paramount. If, on the other hand, the program is closely linked to the proper medication and dosing, such as anticoagulant treatments, then the answer is obvious.

Best practices, the basis for disease management programs, are generally liberal with their medication recommendations. For instance, a clinical practice guideline for heart failure may call for a medication class to be used in a certain situation. The use of an ACE inhibitor, for instance, is beneficial and should be encouraged. In this situation, the disease manager could determine if the person is regularly taking an ACE inhibitor and completely satisfy the guideline; there is no real need to determine dosing. Another classic example of when this level of intervention is appropriate is aspirin use for persons with a prior heart attack. A disease management program consisting of one question to this group, "Are you taking an aspirin every day?", would reap major clinical and financial rewards.

Medication errors, however, are rampant and cause significant morbidity and mortality. The elderly who have complex regimens are especially prone to medication errors. The disease manager must weigh this fact in the decision to, or not to, drill down into greater detail.

If the program requires complete data collection, the best way to frame this part of the conversation is to ask the person if they have already made a list of all their medications with schedule information. If they have, have them read it to you without any other conversation. This exercise becomes one of dictation for a short while. If the person has not done that, ask them to get all their medications and return to the phone. Again, ask them to read them off to you; no other conversation is necessary until you have the list straight. Remember to ask them about *all* medications they take—prescription, alternative, and over-the-counter should all be recorded.

Every disease management program's emphasis on medication information collection varies. The following list is meant to help the manager think through the type of information that may be helpful to know and is presented in order of increasing intensity. Lisinopril is used as an example of a common ACE inhibitor where appropriate.

Medication prescription "Do you have a prescription for the medication?" Although this is usually not the first question on anyone's list, it will be a good question if you discover that a person is not taking a required medication.

Medication presence "Do you have any Lisinopril in the house?" Again, not usually the first question.

Medication adherence "Do you struggle with remembering to take your medications?" *or* "Do you struggle with remembering to take this medication?" Use the struggle word—it implies real-life situation and does not take on the accusatory nature of forgetting or not paying attention.

Medication knowledge "What is the purpose of this medication?" "How does this medication work?" "Are there any special instructions that come with taking this medication?" It stands to reason that the more the person knows about their medications, the more likely they are to adhere to taking them. At a minimum, they should have at least a short-sentence description of why they take each of their medications ("I take it for my blood pressure").

Medication class "Are you currently taking a medication for your heart called a beta-blocker?" This is the most effective question format. It is a simple question and does not require much investigation. At most, the person may know the name of the medication, requiring the disease manager to group the medication into the class.

Medication name "What is the name of the medication?" Normally, the person will answer with the trade name. Generic names are unpronounceable for many.

Medication dose "What is the dosage? It should be a number like 250 mg." This is sometimes a hard thing for the person to communicate, especially if the dosage is in decimal form or the dosage changes by the day. Some medications, like combination medications, do not list the actual dosages.

Medication instructions "How do you take this medication?" You are looking for several parts in this response: the number of pills and the frequency of administration. Some persons have a hard time communicating this to you. Saying "I take two pills twice a day" is hard for some. Repeat it back to them for confirmation.

Medication reactions "Do you have any trouble with this medication?" This is a deep and almost impossible question to rectify from a disease manager's position. Except in the simplest situations (monotherapy with a well-known adverse reaction profile), this detective work is best left to the prescriber. It would be a shame to ascribe an adverse reaction to a critical medication when it wasn't so.

Nonprescription medications "What other medications do you take? Something that you have purchased?" Over-the-counter medications and all manner of alternative medications fall into this category and open up interesting insight into the person's approach to their health. Be careful not to encourage them while they are giving you the list; be nonjudgmental.

Drug–drug interactions Normally, this system is derived from a commercially available medication databases. There are different levels of drug–drug interactions but some are more harmful than others. Physicians may be aware that they have prescribed a drug that has a known conflict and know that it will not do any harm. Many, however, are not aware. Even if the disease manager is a pharmacist, the best reaction to a known drug–drug interaction is to notify the physician and possibly send the person back to them for clarification.

There are common drug–drug interactions that the disease manager should know. Here are the top 10 for the elderly population:

1. Warfarin—NSAIDs
2. Warfarin—Sulfa drugs
3. Warfarin—Macrolides
4. Warfarin—Quinolones
5. Warfarin—Phenytoin
6. ACE inhibitors—Potassium supplements
7. ACE inhibitors—Spironolactone
8. Digoxin—Amiodarone
9. Digoxin—Verapamil
10. Theophylline—Quinolones

Drug–condition interaction A drug–condition interaction is also derived from commercially available medication databases. These interactions tend to be a bit more serious and require redirection back to the prescriber.

Medication regime appropriateness The presence or absence of a medication that falls within a drug class is the hallmark of determining the medical appropriateness of a medication regime. All disease managers should have a feel for the expected medication pattern of the population. When there is a question about whether the person is taking the right medications, there are two common strategies: (1) direct physician communication of the issue and (2) prompting the person to return to the physician to reevaluate their medications.

The primary instruction in this is not to assume that the physician is in error. Medications are prescribed in multiple locations, and there is rarely a common medication database to which to refer.

Polypharmacy evaluation Once there are more than four to five medications, the risk of drug–drug conflicts and self-administration error are high. Pharmacist disease managers excel in this area. Other disease managers should maintain a high sensitivity to the number of medications, complexity of the regimen, and mental capacity of the person when considering the presence of polypharmacy.

Medication seeking and abuse Finding and acting upon a person who is abusing medications is a difficult, but possible, situation. Some disease management programs feature database queries designed for this purpose. Once identified, specially trained disease managers contact both the abuser and their prescribers to open the dialogue.

Without the algorithms, the disease manager is left to discern medication seeking and abuse behavior through conversation. Rare is the disease manager who can identify medication abuse. The common tip-offs are the presence of chronic pain, multiple psychiatric conditions, multiple prescribers, and narcotic or mood-altering medications.

Alternative medication use "What else do you take?" This question can result in a laundry list of preparations that range from daily vitamins to rare and exotic herbs that may be unknown to the disease manager.

Because most disease managers are trained traditionally, knowledge in this area may be lacking. Separate alternative drug references are available and quite helpful. Most alternative medications suffer from the same attributes; they are not developed under FDA clinical trials, are not consistent in their preparation and composition, and most importantly, are not that well understood with respect to their actions with other medications or conditions.

That said, alternative medications are a multibillion dollar business, so it is fair to say that many persons with chronic illness take them. The disease manager should know the top 10 alternative medications and understand the potential interactions and cautions with each.

Problem List

Some disease management programs require the disease manager to complete a problem list. The problem list may be prepopulated with medical utilization files or may have to be manually entered to start. If the list is prepopulated, it may contain either the short or long name of the ICD-9 code.

The challenge for the disease manager is to reconcile this list with the person and to be careful to avoid adding conditions that have not been diagnosed or to remove diagnoses that are real. For instance, persons with heart failure are often not told they have the condition, and when asked, will deny they have the condition.

The purpose of the problem list in many disease management programs is two-fold. First, the list provides a snapshot of the person's medical status. Second, the list may drive the disease manager to do something. Whatever the reason, having some facsimile of a problem list close to hand during the interactions is helpful. The caution here is not to dwell on this list, rather make sure it is understood and accurate.

Try these questions:

"Do you have any chronic conditions?"

"Do you have any conditions that you take medication for?"

"What has the doctor told you about your diagnosis?"

One of the most difficult aspects of the problem list is the requirement to ascribe a status to the condition. If this is a requirement, be very careful in this area. If the person tells you that their condition is under control, qualify that statement with back-up clinical status questions before changing the status to "in control."

Utilization

Some disease management programs are fortunate enough to have daily or regular utilization data that flows into their clinical information system. This data is normally extracted from authorization data in utilization management systems. If this is the case, there is a strong case for acting and prioritizing the presence of an admission or emergency room (ER) visit for a timely encounter.

The disease manager uses this information to determine the person's precipitating events and discharge plan for each event. A large percentage of admissions and ER visits are avoidable, and this represents a major opportunity for the disease manager to intervene at a teachable moment.

Here is a set of questions that will elicit useful information:

"What were the reasons for your visit?"

"What caused you to come to the hospital or ER?"

"What happened when you were there?"

"What did you learn about your condition while you were there?"

"Did they find anything you didn't know before?"

"What did they tell you to do as you were leaving?"

"Do you have a new set of instructions now?"

"Do you have plans to visit your doctor about this visit?"

ASSESSMENT

All disease management programs have some form of assessment. The attributes of assessments are covered in Chapter 8. The purpose of the assessment is to collect clinical data in a standard format. In a research venue, this would be called structured interviewing. The assessment portion of the interaction should feel conversational, free flowing, and helpful.

There are several important dynamics to consider while conducting an assessment. First, for efficiency and effective reasons, introduce the assessment. Start with, "I would like to find out more about what is happening with you. I have a 12-question assessment that will be extremely helpful to both of us." Doing this draws a conceptual line in the conversation, sets a goal of completing 12 questions, and has the effect of getting through the assessment before anything else happens. If the telephone call strays from the initial purpose, the assessment portion is a prime culprit. Keeping the person on track is difficult to do in some cases. The disease manager should focus the person back to the task and complete the 12 questions.

If the assessment is much longer than 15 questions, it will seem extremely long to the person. In these cases, it is paramount to introduce the assessment in the same way, but offer words of encouragement during the assessment. For instance, say "We are half way there. You are really doing a great job with your answers."

Concentrate on the response, not the question. Consider this question and response set, in two scenarios, with two inefficient conversations first:

Disease manager: "First question: I examine my feet for red spots or infection Every day, occasionally, rarely, or never."

Another inefficient conversation goes this way:

Disease manager: "How often do you examine your feet?"

Person: "Sometimes I do. I used to look at them almost every day. Lately, I have been looking at them more carefully. I have a friend who lost a foot recently because of an infection. That scared me. I looked at them yesterday, and the day before, so—sometimes."

Which response does the disease manager choose? How valid would the answer be during data analysis? The answers are not sure and not very.

The more efficient scenario goes like this:

Disease manager: "How often do you examine your feet? Every day, occasionally, rarely, or never? Which one is the best answer?"

Person: "Rarely."

The urge to teach during an assessment is almost insurmountable. Disease managers often use a point brought up while conducting an assessment as a teaching point. Although there is some merit to this approach, problems with this technique also exist. Foremost, the assessment is designed to capture clinical data to drive the next steps, care planning, and caregiving. Until and unless the assessment is complete, this will be difficult to do in a comprehensive fashion.

Second, interjecting teaching points during an assessment may bias subsequent responses. The person may not be forthcoming with the true information if they think that they will get a lecture with a response that doesn't fit the picture of health.

Here are two scenarios; the first one is not recommended:

Disease manager: "Do you use tobacco in any form?"

Person: "Yes, I smoke cigars after I eat. On the porch."

Disease manager: "I'm sure you are aware that cigars carry risks for oral cancer. Some people don't realize this."

Here is the recommended approach:

Disease manager: "Do you use tobacco in any form?"

Person: "Yes, I smoke cigars after I eat. On the porch."

Disease manager: "OK, thanks. Are you in the habit of exercising every day?"

Third, interjecting a teaching point in the middle of an assessment may prove to be a moot point due to an incomplete understanding. More than one disease manager has begun teaching on looking for red spots on the feet during this question, only to find out that the person was vision impaired. This information may have been available within the next several questions.

CARE PLANNING AND CAREGIVING

Once all clinical data is collected, the care planning process can begin. Some of the more sophisticated disease management programs have preset care planning rules. These rules are derived from best practices and are presented to the disease manager as the care plan. Usually, the program will rely on a combination of preset care plans, provided by the program designer and the disease manager's clinical judgment. The format of the care plan may be condition or person centric. Because the majority of disease management programs are condition based, the care plans are as well. It is not unusual to have a separate care plan for diabetes, hypertension, and asthma. The obvious drawback of this approach is that there will certainly be redundant elements in the care plans.

A person centric care plan is agnostic of the conditions and instead presents the elements in a central location. In this case, the redundant elements are removed. Although this sounds far better, and it is, this is an unusual and rare feature. Creating a truly person centric, thus unique, care plan means creating a clinical reasoning-based expert system requiring extensive rule sets and a world-class technical development staff. This ideal is not far away given recent advances.

In the meantime, the disease manager's challenge is to present the care plan in a way that makes sense to the person. Care planning is not creating a course over the telephone, it is a prioritized list of issues to problem solve with the person. The format of the care planning intervention should have at a minimum a name, status, and a mechanism to record progress. Other care planning elements can include goal setting, note taking, and reference materials.

An example of a care planning element follows:

Name: Ensure foot health

Status: Active

Progress: In progress

Goal: Mr. Jones will be able to describe why it is important to examine his feet every day.

Goal status: Not met

Note: Mr. Jones will read the material sent to him and tell me how he is doing on the next phone call.

The caregiving portion of the interaction occurs once the care planning is completed. Optimal program delivery results in disease managers devoting more than half of their time to caregiving. The purpose of caregiving is to act on issues that are negatively affecting health and encouraging health-promoting behaviors.

Caregiving closely matches the care plan, but is not limited to what is written in the care plan. Providing medication knowledge or discussing ways to speak to the doctor are all caregiving activities. Disease managers take note of each of these conversations in progress-note format.

Caregiving can take many forms. In addition to telephonic interaction, disease management programs also use the mail, the Internet, home visits, classes, or clinic visits as mechanisms for delivering messages. The research on the relative effectiveness of each of these modalities is scarce and inconclusive at this time. Common sense would say that each person will respond and react in different ways to the same mechanism, so it may be prudent to deliver the care in a variety of ways.

The last major part of the telephonic interaction is scheduling the next call. If the call went well (defined as both parties feel like they have benefited from the time), the next call is easy to schedule. Because not every call has the same perceived value, it is helpful to begin by introducing the subject of the next call in a positive way and with a sense of excitement: "I can't wait to talk to you about your next steps. I think I can help you feel much better. What time can I call you next week?" This statement engenders true interest and a passion for bettering the health of the person and provides anticipation for the next call.

If the person seems resistant to speaking again, mention that they seem resistant and ask why. Knowing these issues can help resolve problems, provide critical feedback, and ensure more helpful calls in the future.

The telephonic disease management process is extremely challenging and is difficult to master quickly. The goals of both parties are to improve the health status without the benefit of sight or feel.

CHALLENGE QUESTIONS

1. What are some ways a disease manager can convince the person that they are not a telemarketer?
2. Are disease managers prepared to do telephonic work based on their clinical experience?
3. Should a disease manager teach during an assessment or when collecting medication information?

Hospital-Based Disease Management

OVERVIEW

Hospital-based disease management has been around for a long time. These programs have survived through the years because they have worked for patients and their providers of care. There is a wide array of variations on a theme: programs affected by professional orientation—nursing, pharmacist, and physician led; and programs organized by clinical issue—condition based, procedure based, and rehabilitation based.

The purpose of this chapter is to highlight the role of the disease manager within the context of hospital-based disease management. Generally, disease managers are responsible for the application and coordination of clinical standards across hospital staff setting and disciplines. Clinical pathways, which were popularized in the mid-1980s and are still in existence today, were a first attempt at disease management. Clinical pathways are a time-dependent clinical guideline that is separated by either function or discipline. Patient care could be coordinated and critical elements of the guideline were accounted for, but for the most part, clinical pathways were found to be too restrictive. They did not account for the effect of patient status, comorbidities, and human response.

STANDARDS GOVERNING HOSPITAL-BASED
DISEASE MANAGEMENT

Hospitals, by their nature, are highly regulated entities. The Joint Commission Accreditation of Healthcare Organization (JCAHO) has established Standards for Disease-Management Program Certification. The following text provides insight into the nature of hospital-based disease management and is excerpted from the JCAHO accreditation manual:

> JCAHO, the primary hospital accreditation agency, offers a disease-specific certification program with an independent, comprehensive evaluation of organizations that provide a structured program of services for the benefit of participants with specific diseases and conditions. The JCAHO evaluates programs and services under the Disease-Specific Certification Program for two types of organizations:
>
> * organizations that provide clinical care directly to participants. Examples of these organizations include, but are not limited to, hospitals, clinics, home care agencies, long-term care facilities, rehabilitation centers, and physician groups.
> * organizations that provide clinical support and interact directly with participants by telephone or through online services or other electronic resources. Examples of these organizations include, but are not limited to, disease management service organizations and health plans with disease management services.

The standards for the JCAHO disease management certification program are displayed in Table 6.1.

GUIDELINE-BASED DISEASE MANAGEMENT

Clinical practice guidelines are the primary design element of hospital disease management. The guideline will call for patient selection, assessment, treatment choices, and follow-up. The disease manager plays a role in applying this guideline. The following sections provide examples of how this process works in the prehospital phase.

Acute Myocardial Infarction Disease Management

In the pre-hospital phase, the disease manager will ensure[1]:

* Availability of 911 access.
* Availability of an emergency medical services (EMS) system staffed by persons trained to treat cardiac arrest with defibrillation if indicated and to triage patients with ischemic-type chest discomfort.

Table 6.1   JCAHO Disease Management Standards

DF1	Practitioners are qualified and competent.
DF2	The program uses a standardized process originating in clinical guidelines or evidence-based practice to deliver or facilitate the delivery of clinical care.
DF3	The program tailors the standardized process to meet the needs of the participant.
DF4	Concurrently occurring conditions are managed or the information necessary for their management is communicated to the appropriate practitioner(s).
DF5	The standardized process is revised or improved through the ongoing collection and evaluation of data regarding variance from the clinical practice guidelines.
PM1	The program uses measurement data to evaluate process and outcomes.
PM2	The program uses information from measurement data to support, improve, or validate clinical decision making.
PM3	Participant-specific, care-related data is captured, calculated, analyzed, and, as appropriate, reported.
PM4	Participant perception of quality of care (satisfaction) is evaluated.
PM5	Data quality and integrity are maintained.
SE1	The program involves participants in making decisions about the management of their diseases or conditions.
SE2	The program addresses lifestyle changes that support self-management regimens.
SE3	The program addresses participants' education needs.
PR1	The program has an organized, comprehensive approach to performance improvement.
PR2	Leadership roles in the program are clearly defined.
PR3	The program is relevant for the targeted population or health care service areas.

Table 6.1   JCAHO Disease Management Standards (*continued*)

PR4	The scope and level of care or services offered by the program are provided to participants.
PR5	Eligible patients have access to the care or services provided by the program.
PR6	The scope and level of care or services provided are comparable for individuals with the same acuity and type of condition.
PR7	The program's leaders and, as appropriate, participants, practitioners, and community leaders collaborate to design, implement, and evaluate services.
PR8	The program complies with applicable laws and regulations.
PR9	The program operates in an ethical manner.
PR10	Facilities where participants receive care are safe and physically accessible.
PR11	The program has reference and resource materials readily available.
PR12	The process for identifying, reporting, managing, and tracking unanticipated, untoward adverse events is defined and implemented.
CT1	The confidentiality and security of participant information is preserved.
CT2	The program gathers information about the participant's disease or condition from practitioners and settings across the continuum of care.
CT3	The program shares information about the participant's disease or condition across the entire continuum of care to any relevant setting or practitioner.
CT4	Information management processes meet the program's internal and external information needs.
CT5	The program initiates, maintains, and makes accessible a health or medical record for every participant.

Source: Delivering or Facilitating Clinical Care. In: *Disease-Specific Care Certification Manual Standards Chapters,* 2002, pp. 23–26. Joint Commission Accreditation of Healthcare Organizations, Oakbrook Terrace, IL.

- Availability of a first-responder defibrillation program in a tiered response system.
- Health care providers to educate patients and families about signs and symptoms of acute myocardial infarction (MI), accessing EMS, and medications.
- Twelve-lead telemetry.
- Prehospital thrombolysis in special circumstances (e.g., transport time greater than 90 minutes).

The disease manager will put an education plan in place that identifies persons with known heart disease in affiliated clinics or through physicians who have privileges to the hospital. Once identified, the patients will:

1. Be educated by physicians, nurses, and staff about common symptoms of acute myocardial infarction and appropriate actions to take after symptom onset.
2. Be given an action plan that covers: (1) the prompt use of aspirin and nitroglycerin if available, (2) how to access EMS, and (3) the location of the nearest hospital that offers 24-hour emergency cardiac care.
3. Be given a copy of their resting ECG as a baseline to aid physicians in the emergency department.
4. Emphasize the importance of acting promptly. Family members should be included in these discussions and enlisted as advocates for action when symptoms of infarction are apparent.

FOLLOW-UP–BASED DISEASE MANAGEMENT

Stroke Follow-up

The disease manager may also devise a program that is designed to ensure appropriate follow-up of persons recently hospitalized for stroke. The disease manager will put mechanisms in place to identify in-patient stroke patients about to be discharged, develop educational materials, and devise home visits and other follow-up mechanisms.

PROCEDURE-BASED DISEASE MANAGEMENT

The disease manager in the cardiac catheritization lab designs and implements a program that provides preprocedure checklists, education, and counseling. After the procedure, the disease manager contacts the patient to ensure appropriate healing and that post-procedure symptoms are minimized.

CONDITION-BASED SELF-CARE DISEASE MANAGEMENT

Condition-based self-care disease management programs provide an opportunity for the disease manager to speak or interact with more than one patient at a time. Typically, the subject matter focuses on the practical aspects of self-care and encourages the participants to share their thoughts, tips, and challenges relative to their condition.

For instance, the disease manager, in concert with hospital-based clinics, organizes a program for diabetics that includes written material, classes on diabetes basics, nutrition, exercise, insulin therapy, foot care, and blood glucose monitoring. In addition, the disease manager coordinates teaching by a podiatrist, registered dietician, ophthalmologist, internal medicine doctor, and certified diabetes educator. The program also offers a once-a-month diabetes support group.

CHALLENGE QUESTIONS

1. From what hospital department might a disease manager come?
2. Why would a hospital support disease management? What is in it for them?

Endnotes

1. Ryan, T.J., Antman, E.M., Brooks, N.H., Califf, R.M., Hillis, L.D., Hiratzka, L.F., et al. *ACC/AHA guidelines for the management of patients with acute myocardial infarction.* 1999 update: A report of the American College of Cardiology/American Heart Association Task Force on Practice Guidelines (Committee on Management of Acute Myocardial Infarction). Available at *www.acc.org.* Accessed on April, 2004.

Clinical Basis for Disease Management

OVERVIEW

Every disease management program starts with a clinical foundation. In a sense, a disease management program is the application of clinical knowledge that has been distilled into easily digestible parts, then reformulated to improve a patient's health status. Program designers comb the research literature and use practice guidelines to ensure the integrity of the clinical reasoning and resulting messaging. Disease managers use this information set to guide them in their interactions with their patients.

This chapter will unravel the path of clinical information as it weaves its way through disease management program design. The chapter will also provide methods for the disease manager to use the clinical foundations to measure the impact of the program.

EVIDENCE-BASED MEDICINE

Evidence-based medicine (EBM) is a common and often misunderstood term used in disease management. David Sackett and associates, well-respected experts in the EBM field, define evidence-based medicine as "the conscientious, explicit, and judicious use of current best evidence in making decisions about the care of individual patients."[1] The degree to which current best evidence varies depends greatly on the disease state or treatment modality.

EBM is not a rigid set of guidelines written to provide absolutely perfect care. EBM depends on the human elements of clinical expertise, compassion, empathy, and discernment in order for it to be applied in a judicious manner. Decision making is at the heart of EBM and that is why the first imperative is to know all about the patient. In order to apply the simplest EBM, the disease manager must understand the hopes and fears, social aspects, coping mechanisms, and community resources of the person and also have an awareness of the desired treatment goals. Without this backdrop, EBM is useless.

Consider this application of EBM. We know from the literature that taking a 80 mg aspirin is effective in reducing the incidence of a second heart attack. This statement is straight out of the literature and does not mean that all people who use an aspirin will avoid a second heart attack. The patient may have a preexisting disease that is so severe that an aspirin won't work, or there may be significant peptic ulcer disease that prevents the use of aspirin altogether. In this way, EBM is a good starting point but may never make it inside the care plan.

When present, EBM provides clinical anchors upon which disease managers can begin their interventions. Reliance on EBM prevents the variety of opinions that are bound to arise during a clinical situation. Disease managers can always hang on to the evidence and go from there. If there is not a reliable EBM source, then the disease manager is left with the best approximation of the truth, often having to combine clinical impression, facts, and past experience.

One of the most powerful aspects of EBM is that it inevitably changes and improves itself over time. The EBM in the late 1990s called for a diabetes diagnosis to be made with a blood glucose value of 140 mg/dl or above on more than one occasion. Now it has been lowered to 126 mg/dl on 2 separate days, and on the day that research was published, there were many more diabetics in the world. On the negative side, because EBM changes and physicians may not be aware of the changes, the quality of care suffers.

There have been many studies to demonstrate that the knowledge of EBM dramatically declines in as little as 5 years after medical school. In one example, a study by Anne Stephenson and colleagues[2] found that only 50 percent of family practice physicians felt comfortable recognizing melanoma, a highly dangerous and lethal skin cancer. In this study, the physicians were well aware that melanoma was dangerous, but could not recount the risk factors or clinical attributes of the lesion. This is one of many examples why disease managers are critical in helping the patient stay on top of medical issues on which they cannot necessarily depend on their doctor.

EBM is not a mindless application of research. Instead, the disease manager should decide whether the EBM applies to the patient, then discuss the options. This implies that EBM is best practiced in a dynamic environment where the disease manager poses clinically sound questions, uses research to reason out the responses, then combines knowledge of the patient with the EBM to arrive at a conclusion.

The ultimate application of EBM is in the formation of the clinical question. The question must consider the patient, the intervention, an alternative intervention, and the evidence. Here is a short scenario that illustrates this process.

Thelma, an elderly black woman, is taking Verapamil, a calcium channel blocker, for her hypertension. She states that she notices that her home blood pressure readings are consistently greater than 140/90. She is having adverse reactions and wonders if there might be a more effective medication for her.

Broken down, this scenario looks like this:

Patient and situation: Elderly, black with hypertension with adverse reactions

Present intervention: Verapamil

EBM interventions: ACE inhibitors, diuretics, or beta blockers

Desired outcome: Improve blood pressure with most effective medication

This information comes together to form the question, "What is the most effective blood pressure medication class for elderly, black women?"

The evidence points to:

1. There is no apparent difference in treatment efficacy across racial groups.

Though many articles have been written about the varied effects of blood pressure medications on various ethnic or racial groups, many of these generalizations do not apply to individuals. It is better to apply the principles of pharmacologic therapy described elsewhere in this article rather than base treatment on ethnic or racial considerations.[3]

2. A combination of a low dose diuretic and beta blocker is effective.

The SHEP trial showed that low-dose diuretic therapy, with beta-blockers added as a second step if needed, reduces the incidence of stroke and coronary events in elderly persons with hypertension. The benefits of therapy occur in patient with and without diabetes.[4]

This exercise may seem arduous, but when done once and duplicated across many patients, it is an extremely efficient and sure method to apply evidence-based medicine. In this example, the research was of the highest order.

RESEARCH PYRAMID

Times exist when the research is less rigorous. The notion of ever-increasing levels of research is best described using the research pyramid that is used to measure the efficacy of treatments. The pyramid (see Figure 7.1) is presented inverted to illustrate the topmost level of research rigor. For the most part, EBM is confined to the top three designs because the studies in these designs return results that point to the most credible results due to randomized sample selection, controlling for extraneous variables, and the increased likelihood that the results are not as a result of chance.

Figure 7.1   Research Pyramid

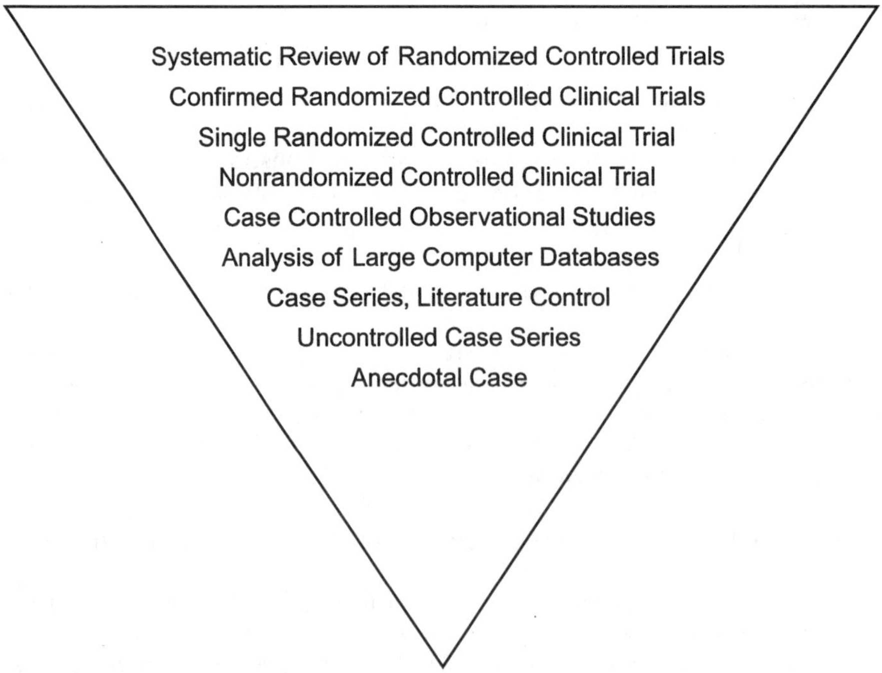

Systematic Review of Randomized Controlled Trials
Confirmed Randomized Controlled Clinical Trials
Single Randomized Controlled Clinical Trial
Nonrandomized Controlled Clinical Trial
Case Controlled Observational Studies
Analysis of Large Computer Databases
Case Series, Literature Control
Uncontrolled Case Series
Anecdotal Case

PROGRAM OUTCOMES

For the purposes of this explanation, outcomes are defined as the result of the disease management program, obviously of which the disease manager plays a critical role. Disease management programs typically track four kinds of outcomes (subcategories included for illustration purposes):

1. Financial outcomes
   a. Total medical costs
   b. Condition-related costs
   c. Costs by place of service
   d. Cost trend from start of program
2. Clinical outcomes
   a. Clinical exam rates
   b. Lab values
   c. Symptom severity
   d. Knowledge cases
3. Quality of life outcomes
   a. Functional status
   b. Perception of general health status
4. Satisfaction outcomes
   a. Patient
   b. Physician
   c. Disease management program sponsor

Financial Outcomes

Financial outcomes are normally taken from medical and pharmacy claims data. Health claims are generated when a physician renders care and presents a "claim" to the health plan. The most interesting parts of a claim to the disease manager are the date, place of service, ICD-9 or CPT code, and amount paid for services.

Some question exists about the validity of the ICD-9 code on a claim because there is no reliable quality assurance mechanism in place to ensure that the claim truly reflects the work done. This is primarily a large honor system and one that is unfortunately an important aspect of the financial outcomes. One is left with the law of averages; there is a constant rate of over- and underbilling, so differences in pre- and post-financial costs contain the same error.

Financial outcomes are calculated in a dizzying array of methods to accommodate for medical inflation, medical spending trends, and regression to the mean. Suffice it to say that tracking and reporting financial outcomes is best left to those who are experts in health claims data analysis and accounting. The final result is expressed as a savings percentage or a return on investment. The value proposition chapter (see Chapter 4) explains how this is calculated in more detail. The following example illustrates how a disease management program could demonstrate savings using a cost avoidance model.

The cost avoidance financial model is based on the premise that medical expenses increase at a certain rate. The 2004 forecasted inflation rate is 14.8 percent (see Table 7.1). That means that if there was nothing done to intervene with a population, their costs would rise 14.8 percent.

When a disease management program is introduced to higher cost patients, the cost increase trend would be slowed. In Table 7.2, the 14.8 percent medical inflation factor is applied to a population that had a $1 million increase in their medical costs, but the inflation rate was slowed to prevent the expected $2.5 million increase. One can say that because of the disease management intervention (and a lot of good work by disease managers), the inflation rate was slowed to 4 percent for this group.

Clinical Outcomes

Clinical outcomes are considered process outcomes because they address issues that lead to utilizing health resources. Clinical outcomes can be subjective or objective. Examples of subjective clinical outcomes include:

Self-reported pain scale rating

Adherence to medications

Smoking rates

Use of blood glucose meter

Table 7.1   2004 Forecasted Medical Inflation Rates

Model	Inflation Trend in %
HMO	14.8
POS	14.8
PPO	14.9
Indemnity	16.3

Table 7.2   Medical Inflation Trend and Savings Calculation

			Inflation Adjusted Trended Costs	Difference Considering the Inflation Rate
Medical Inflation Trend	14.8%			
	Year Prior to Program	**1 Year After 1st Year**		
Total Medical Costs	$24,345,790	$25,365,788	$27,948,966.92	$2,583,179
Actual Cost Difference	$1,019,998			
Savings	9%			
New Medical Inflation Rate with Disease Management Program	4%			

Adequate peak flow meter technique

Ability to respond to a hypoglycemic reaction

Self-reported home blood glucose meter readings

Examples of objective clinical outcomes are:

Lab values

Blood pressure, pulse, weight (clinician observed)

Any clinician-to-patient observation

Clinical outcomes arise from the EBM portion of the program design. The evidence will point to certain key clinical data or facts that when known should help an astute disease manager arrive at the best care option. The EBM for heart failure clearly points to needing to track daily weights to make judgments about fluid status. At least two clinical outcomes come from this: the presence of a daily weigh log and the number of patients who weigh themselves daily. Disease managers concentrate on clinical process outcomes such as these because if they are not addressed, then getting to the clinical and financial value proposition is much more difficult.

From a statistical standpoint, clinical outcomes cover the entire spectrum of data types and are measured in different ways. Refer to Table 7.3 to see why this is so.

Continuous Data is in the form of numbers and is continuous to infinity.

Ordinal Data is in the form of numbers that have a logical order and are expressed as a scale.

Interval Data is composed of discreet values such as a five-point scale which contains values from 1 to 5 and represents a description. Lickert scales produce interval data by assigning a 1 to very rarely, a 2 to rarely, a 3 to occasionally, and so forth.

Nominal Data is in the form of words such as rarely, occasionally, and always. Nominal data has no logical order.

Binary Data is limited to two values: yes or no; present or absent.

Tracking and measuring clinical outcomes is in the purview of the program manager and a credible health research statistician. The disease manager may not feel like they are in a research program, but in many ways they are. This is why the quality of data capture and adherence to the program design is important.

Quality of Life Outcomes

Quality of life outcomes are measured using validated surveys such as the SF-12 or Minnesota Living with Heart Failure surveys. These and similar surveys are meant to quantify the quality of life from a variety of domains. Using the SF-12 as an example, the test measures across subdomains that are general health, physical functioning, role functioning (physical), bodily pain, vitality, role functioning (emotional), mental health, and social functioning.

The SF-12 results are presented by subdomain and can be compared to matched groups or can be compared to a prior testing period. Like any test that measures qualitative parameters, it has inherent limitations. The contribution of the SF-12 and other similar surveys to disease management and to disease management practice is in evolution. For most programs, the SF-12 is used as one measure of impact, but is not used to drive specific interventions. Low scores in the bodily pain subdomain could influence a more robust pain reduction intervention, for instance.

Table 7.3   Clinical Outcome Data Types and Measurement

Clinical Outcome	Data Type*	Measurement
Weight	Continuous	t-test—independent means
Pain rating using a 1–10 scale	Ordinal	Mann-Whitney U test, Wilcoxon or Sign test, Friedman's AOV by ranks, Kruskal-Wallis AOV, Spearman's rank order correlation, Kendall's Tau
Quality of life using a five-point Lickert scale	Interval	t-test—independent means, t-test—dependent (nonindependent) means, interrupted time-series analysis, repeated measures analysis of variance *or* analysis of co-variance, analysis of variance, one-group t-test, Kolmogorov-Smirnov test for goodness-of-fit, Pearson product moment correlation coefficient
Medical history of certain conditions	Nominal	Chi-square, McNemar test, Cochran's Q, Chi-square test for K independent groups, Chi-square goodness-of-fit test, Lambda Beta, Phi coefficient
Active tobacco user (Yes/No)	Binary	Descriptive statistics, frequency table, Rates

*Data Types

Satisfaction Outcomes

Satisfaction outcome surveys are given to patients and physicians and are normally conducted by external agencies. Disease management programs use the results to quantify the overall acceptance of the program in terms of perceived usefulness and effectiveness. Typically, patient satisfaction scores average in the 85 to 95 percent range (mostly or very satisfied) and physicians' scores average somewhat lower. The current physician satisfaction issues are the multiplicity of disease management programs across their patients, their lack of understanding of the benefit of disease management, and low rates of survey completion.

TYING IT ALL TOGETHER

The purpose of this chapter is to lay out the clinical components and measurement of a disease management program. Figure 7.2 illustrates the relative influence and integration of each of these components.

Disease management practice is the sum of incorporating patient characteristics, formulating the clinical question, crafting an optimal intervention, and delivering that intervention to the patient in a way that positively affects financial and clinical outcomes. Doing this requires a sound EBM foundation, the flexibility to consider the patient, and the ability to synthesize the information into a workable intervention.

Because disease management practice is relatively new, the overall quality of clinical integrity of the process is widely varied. Multiple pieces need to come together to ensure the highest quality practice. These pieces include clear program expectations, the best EBM available, excellent disease manager training, state-of-the-art clinical information systems, and an operational infrastructure that is tailored to the volume and intensity of the targeted population.

Figure 7.2   Integration of Clinical Components

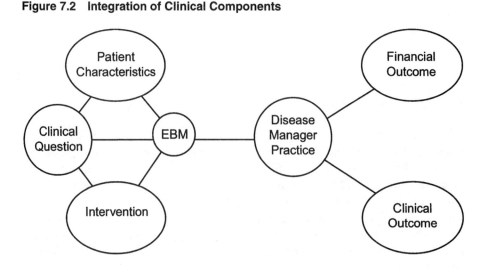

CHALLENGE QUESTIONS

1. What is the relationship between financial and clinical outcomes? Does one always lead to the other?

2. What additional skills does a disease manager need to have to formulated an evidence-based clinical question?

3. What are some of the environmental challenges present when measuring financial and clinical outcomes?

Endnotes

1. Sackett, D. L., W. S. Richardson, W. Rosenberg. *Clinical Epidemiology: A Basic Science for Clinical Medicine*, 2nd ed. Boston: Little, Brown, 1991.

2. Stephenson, A. From L. Cohen and J. Tipping, "Family Physicians' Knowledge of Malignant Melanoma." *Journal of the American Academy of Dermatology* 37, no. 6 (December 1997).

3. Calvert, J. *Clinics in Family Practice*, vol. 3, no. 4. Philadelphia: W. B. Saunders Company, 2001.

4. Systolic Hypertension in the Elderly Program (SHEP) Cooperative Research Group. "Prevention of Stroke by Antihypertensive Drug Treatment in Older Persons with Isolated Systolic Hypertension: Final Results of SHEP." *Journal of the American Medical Association* 265 (1991): 3255–3364 and The Treatment of Mild Hypertension Research Group. "The Treatment of Mild Hypertension Study: A Randomized, Placebo-Controlled Trial of a Nutritional-Hygienic Regimen Along with Various Drug Monotherapies." *Archives of Internal Medicine* 151 (1991): 1413–1423.

Developing a Disease Management Program

OVERVIEW

There are times when a disease manager is asked to develop or participate in the development of a new program. This chapter covers the major tasks involved in constructing a program and is not meant to be exhaustive. A full treatment of this subject is a book unto its own.

All programs do not have the same components. Program development will be heavily dependent on the setting, value proposition, funding, human resources, and available technology. The best way to develop a disease management program is to begin with the value proposition—covered in Chapter 4. Once this is clearly understood and agreed upon, program development is much easier.

MEMBER IDENTIFICATION

The first step in program development is to determine who is in and who is out of the program. This task is not as easy as it seems. If the source data is reliable—and it sometimes is not—things are easier. The primary problem with

71

questionable data is the amount of false positives (persons who should not be included in the group) and false negatives (persons who the identification has missed). Disease managers feel this effect; when they are making contact with the wrong people, the discussion can become difficult.

There are several common targeting strategies worth mentioning. Rules-based targeting is by far the most common method used in disease management. An example of a rules-based identification algorithm is shown in Chapter 4. In this method, rules are developed that are used to identify the population. Typically, rules are in the form of ICD-9, CPT, or other similar medical claims codes. Other rules can include age, gender, or lab values. Whatever the source of the rule, be sure that if a person satisfies the rule that they are likely appropriate for the program. As a way of ensuring this happens, consider writing rules that are self-checking. Consider the following rule:

Diabetes Identification Rule 1: Anybody who has an ICD-9 code of 250.0.

This rule is simple enough but this rule will also produce a lot of false positives. This will happen because many times the ICD-9 code 250.0 will be used with a person for whom diabetes is suspected. Whether or not the diabetes was confirmed will be determined on the first contact.

Instead, consider this amended rule:

Diabetes Identification Rule 2: Anybody who has at least four claims on separate days for ICD-9 code 250.0 in the past 6 months.

Introducing two factors, the number of times a claim is present and a time frame of 6 months, creates a higher likelihood of a true diabetes diagnosis. Other factors used to tighten up or narrow the population include age, gender, and place of service.

PREDICTIVE MODELING

In some cases, predictive modeling may be used to identify the population. For the most part, predictive modeling is best applied to programs that are focused on utilization of services with an eye toward reducing unnecessary utilization. The result of predictive modeling is a score, usually a number from zero to one. This allows a population to be rank ordered.

Predictive modeling comes in two varieties: rules based and neural net based. Rules-based predictive modeling uses codes or identifiers that when found in a pattern, predict future utilization for the person. These rules are then applied to standard inferential statistics equations to arrive at the risk score. This is also called regression analysis and is best left to those who have training in biostatisitics. Rules-based predictive models have a 60 percent chance, on average, to accurately predict future utilization. This is 10 percent better than the toss of a coin.

Neural net-based predictive modeling also predicts future utilization and produces a rank-ordered list of persons. The major difference with this kind of predictive modeling is in how the rules relate to one another. Neural models allow for certain factors to be included or excluded based on many factors. It is not unusual to have a predictive model to contain over 100 factors, and only 8 be used in the actual equation after the data is completed. Like the rules-based version, this exercise is best left to those who are trained in this area. Neural net-based predictive modeling is more predictive than strictly rules based. It is possible to achieve an 85 percent accuracy in predicting future utilization.

Some disease management programs contain a trigger or focus list, which contain entrance rules for the program. Health care professionals use a trigger list to identify potential program enrollees. This method has merit in that the persons referred to the program are likely to be prequalified, and appropriate, unlike strictly automatic rules based. The downside of this method is that it depends on persons remembering the list and manually referring them to the program.

The last common, but least used, method of identification is self-referral. Self-referral requires clear entrance criteria and easy-to-understand enrollment instructions. Here is an example message:

> If you have diabetes and are taking insulin, the diabetes wellness program may be just right for you. Call 1-800-333-5555 for more details.

This message includes the rules: diabetic and taking insulin. This helps to ensure that the person has diabetes, and the person has Type 1 or a more advanced Type 2 diabetes. Self-referrals share the same characteristics as the focus list—more reliable confirmation of the condition or engagement rule, but operationally arduous.

CLINICAL CONTENT

Disease managers are stewards of clinical practice guidelines and as such are guided by the best medicine possible. For the major conditions, there are nationally developed guidelines, which are signed, sealed, and approved. Some disease management programs do not have one guideline, but rather several credible sources of medical information from which to draw. Gaps in care, best practices, and intervention strategies are all subjects covered while developing the value proposition. Here they form the clinical content of the program.

Gaps in care become potential program clinical outcomes. Increasing the rate of clinical foot exams for diabetics is an outcome that comes from the literature, which demonstrates that this exam is rarely done. This gap causes morbidity in the late identification of neuropathy and infection, all leading to amputation. Gaps in care also drive program interventions. In this case, the program designer may include a monofiliment testing kit in an introductory mailing.

Clinical content review also drives the kind of data capture required to prompt the disease manager to perform an intervention. Examples of data points include tobacco use, home blood glucose monitoring, exercise, nutrition, and alcohol habits. All of these data points are inserted in the assessment (described in greater detail later in this chapter).

The last major use for clinical content review is decompensation factors. This is probably the most demanding step and most disease management designers glance over it or skip it altogether. A decompensation review combs the literature for factors that produce a worsening of symptoms. One reference may indicate that once they have had their first amputation, more than 50 percent of diabetics will lose the other limb in the next year. This situation points to a decompensation factor that, if known, can create interventions to prevent a worsening situation.

SEGMENTATION

Segmentation is another population identification method used primarily for larger populations and is used in concert with predictive modeling. Segmentation is an automatic sorting of persons into predefined groupings. Usually this sorting occurs after the initial identification and before contact with a disease manager. The outcome of segmentation is a segmented—or bucketed—group of persons. For example, let's say that we have identified 10,000 diabetics who are eligible for a disease management program. Because 10,000 people are difficult to contact at one time, we apply predictive modeling to the population, then divide the group into four segments. Using the predictive model scores, we reserve the top 5 percent of the predictive model scores to the highest group, the next 25 percent to the next group, and the final 70 percent to the following group. This allows for crafting interventions that may be tailored to three different groups before contact begins.

The trick to segmentation is to concentrate on percentiles versus rank order. It is better in the long run to keep the thresholds relative rather than absolute. This way the groups always contain the same acuity level. The component discussed next, stratification, has some relationships with segmentation. Ideally, segmentation and stratification have strong agreement.

STRATIFICATION

Most disease management programs have some form of stratification. Stratification serves three primary purposes: (1) assigning contact intensity, (2) deriving an overall clinical picture, and (3) matching a person to the appropriate disease manager. The components of stratification are clinical in nature and rules based. Generally, stratification occurs as a result of a disease manager assessment or certain clinical data. There are usually three to five strata within a given program. The number of stratification levels depends on many factors, but is usually dependent on an already established number. If the disease management program is newly forming, consider choosing fewer, rather than more, levels. This keeps operational complexity to a minimum.

The mechanics behind stratification are many and are a highly guarded secret for disease management companies. This is because how one parses out the people in the program speaks to the efficiency and effectiveness necessary to impact a large population. The following example describes a general scheme using assessment responses as the basis for stratification.

Stratification example—Diabetes Program
Three stratification levels: 1 is the lowest, 3 the highest
  Level 3
      Blood glucose average for past month > 300mg/dl
      or
      Hba1c greater than 11
      or
      Hospitalized for diabetic control in past 6 months
      or
      Myocardial infarction in past year
      or
      Open wound or active infection
  Level 2
      Type 1 diabetes
      or
      No regular blood glucose monitoring
      or
      Hba1c between 9–11
  Level 1
      All the rest

Using this example, one can see that a Level-3 person will require more intensive follow-up and perhaps a more experienced disease manager. Level-2 persons will require education and support, which will hopefully prevent them from moving to Level-3 status. Level-1 persons will have no significant diabetic issues and may need rare interactions or perhaps just mailed interventions.

One way to think of the value of stratification is clinical decompensation. Especially for the chronically ill populations, the health status direction is almost always to the worse. Stratification is one way to gauge the degree of decompensation; higher acuity people are in a more rapid decline than lower acuity people.

ASSESSMENT

Every disease manager asks questions. Most programs have predetermined assessments. Some assessments are quite rigid in their format, while others are free form. Program designers will fit the assessment format to the overall approach. Large disease management initiatives will tend to have tighter assessment structure; programs that are more intense and will need to accommodate a wide variety of situations have a looser structure. No matter what the program design, there is always a need to ask questions.

There are several overarching principles about assessment design:

- Disease management assessments follow a structured interview format.
- They must be constructed so that the questions can be answered in any order because few assessments are answered in order.
- Assessments are also a data capturing tool that ensure that data is consistently and reliably stored.
- The only real reason for an assessment is to collect responses. Experienced disease managers concentrate on the responses rather than the questions.

Assessment Types

There are three primary assessment formats: form, nested, and branch chain. As stated earlier, the assessment type depends on the data capture requirements.

Form-Based Assessment

A form-based assessment is a simple list of questions and responses. There is no logic within the assessment. The questions and responses are visible in every circumstance. This type of assessment is found in paper-based programs and relatively simple programs. Flexibility and potentially validated data capture are weak points of a form-based assessment. Let's take a look at an example. Comments about each question are in brackets.

Form-Based Assessment
1. What type of diabetes do you have?
   a. Type 1
   b. Type 2
2. What kind of medication do you take for your diabetes?
   a. None
   b. Oral medications
   c. Insulin

[Question 2 is not necessary for the Type 1 diabetic; redundant for this group.]
3. Do you own a blood glucose monitor?
   a. Yes
   b. No

[Simple question, but not a good one for a form-based format.]
4. How often do you check your blood glucose?
   a. Once a day
   b. Once a week
   c. Rarely
   d. Never

[The never answer to this question has two meanings. They may own a monitor and never test, or they never check because they don't own a monitor.]
5. Do you use tobacco?
   a. Yes
   b. No

[Another simple question but getting into trouble again.]
6. How long have you smoked?
   a. Less than 5 years
   b. More than 5 years
   c. Don't smoke

[Response "c" is there because of Question 5. Disease managers hate this unnecessary question after the second time they complete the survey.]
7. [Other questions as needed.]

Nested Assessment

The use of a nested survey is better than a form-based assessment. Questions are enabled based on prior responses or a pattern of responses. The interviewer will still see all the questions and responses, but will not be able to answer questions that are disabled. A short nested assessment demonstrates how this works.

Nested Assessment
1. What is your gender?
    a. Male [Skip to Question 3.]
    b. Female [Continue to Question 2.]
2. Are you considering pregnancy?
    a. Yes [Skip to Question 4.]
    b. No [Skip to Question 4.]
3. Have you had your prostate checked?
    a. Yes [Skip to Question 4.]
    b. No [Continue to Question 4.]
4. How many alcohol drinks do you have in a day?
    a. 1–2
    b. 3–4
    c. More than 4

Branch-Chain Logic Assessment

The branch-chain logic assessment is by far the best format, but is rarely used in a disease management setting. This type of assessment presents its questions and responses one question at a time. The assessment literally builds based on the prior response. Because it is difficult to guide someone through this process, as well as the difficulty in supporting this format technologically, it remains on the shelf waiting innovation.

ASSESSMENT BUILDING

Assessments should be built to be reliable, valid, efficient, and effective. To do this, much thought and attention must be paid to the question order, format of the question, contextual agreement of the question and response, and response types.

In general, questions should be asked in order of general to specific within logical groupings. Here is an example assuming a nested format—logic implied:

1. Do you exercise?
    a. Yes
    b. No
2. How many minutes a day do you exercise?

3. Does this feel like the right amount of minutes to you?
   a. Yes
   b. No

This example starts with a rather general binary question about the presence or absence of exercise and leads to a more specific intensity question, which then leads to an even more specific question about whether the intensity feels right to the person. The next group of questions may start with a general question about sleep patterns, then drill down to other aspects about sleep.

The question format is extremely important. Questions can be in text box, multiple choice, numerical, and date formats. This seems like a fairly simple attribute, but consider this question in date format:

1. Date of the last myocardial infarction [insert date here].

It seems like a good, clean question, but what happens if the person has never had a heart attack? There is no reasonable answer given the format. Be careful when choosing a question format; consider every possibility.

The question-response agreement is probably the most overlooked aspect of assessment building. In short, the question should match the responses in the same context. Here is an example of a question with poor agreement:

1. How would you rate your pain?
   a. Light during the day
   b. Medium when I exercise
   c. Heavy at night

This is a poor question-and-response set. The data from this question is almost useless. Quite often, the assessment builder is trying squeeze out other information in the question, but this doesn't work for a variety of reasons. It is better to cleanly separate the questions into domains. Our poor example had three domains: degree of pain, timing, and activity. This question should really be three questions:

1. How would you rate your pain?
   a. Light
   b. Medium
   c. Heavy
2. When is your pain at its worse? (check all that apply)
   a. Morning
   b. Afternoon
   c. Night
3. Does activity cause pain?
   a. Yes
   b. No

Finally, the response type is a critical component of the assessment and can bring tremendous efficiency gains if done correctly. The usual response types are pick one, pick many, date, integer, decimal, and text. The date, integer, and decimal response types should all have validation parameters to prevent data entry errors. A person should not have a birth date of January 1, 1298, for instance.

CARE PLANNING

The purpose of care planning is to craft a set of interventions. The interventions can take any form and come from anywhere. Care planning is truly an art and a science rolled into one. Crafting intervention implies that there is clinical reasoning that occurs in the process. Some program designs rely heavily on a disease manager to create the care plan, while others have extremely robust clinical-reasoning systems that propose care plans for the disease manager. The degree of sophistication used in care planning is a function of the setting, outcome expectations, and technology to support the program.

Common intervention formats include telephonic encounter, mailed or Web-based reading materials, and in-person encounters in the home or clinic. Each intervention has a cost and an impact all its own. Table 8.1 describes this relationship in general terms.

Care planning also must be flexible enough to meet the needs of the person; that is to say that some persons prefer mail over telephone contact, some are visual learners, and some require a combination of approaches. The disease manager should be sensitive to these attributes in order to reach maximal effectiveness for the care plan.

Table 8.1   Common Disease Management Intervention Formats

Intervention Format	Cost	Impact
Telephonic encounters	Medium	Medium to high
Mailed or Web-based reading materials	Low	Low to medium
In-person encounters	High	High

CAREGIVING

Once care planning elements are in place, the caregiving can begin. Caregiving for disease managers is defined as the act of carrying out the care plan. Like care planning, caregiving can take several formats. The primary mechanisms for disease managers are education, motivational interviewing, and goal setting.

A large percentage of traditional disease management caregiving is education. This is a natural extension of both the heavy reliance on self-management skills, prerequisite knowledge required for self-management, and the profession of the disease manager. Breaking this down a little further, we can readily appreciate the need for a diabetic to know why blood glucose control is necessary, understand how to monitor the blood glucose, and receive this instruction from a dietician, pharmacist, or nurse.

MOTIVATIONAL INTERVIEWING

Motivational interviewing is critical to the success of caregiving. Disease managers who are successful share the ability to motivate, encourage, and otherwise prod a person to do the right thing for their health's sake. Unfortunately, training in this area is sparse to nonexistent. There are many texts on motivational speaking, persuasion, and selling, but almost none that speak directly on this subject. The best work in this area comes from www.motivatehealthyhabits.com, a body of work produced by Richard J. Botelho, a medical doctor from the University of Rochester in New York. Dr. Botelho provides a series of books on this subject, as well as Web-based training. A list of excellent readings on this topic can be found in the reference section.

The main tenets for motivational interviewing include active listening, recognizing and affirming that the person has real issues and barriers, gently and carefully pointing out current health actions and desire for goals, and instilling hope for better things through positive language and encouraging the person to use change-related language.

Goal setting is the last caregiving technique. Although this may seem like an easy thing to do, seasoned disease managers know how difficult this can be for some. Writing a goal can be an intimidating step in the caregiving process, and some people may not be ready for it. Most people don't have written goals—they have thoughts, dreams, and aspirations. Goal setting, however, is a powerful tool when done correctly.

The process of initiating and setting a goal is not standard, but there are common elements that should be considered, and the design should make accommodations for them.

1. Consider the language leading up to a goal. Say, "Would you like to work on quitting smoking?" or "How would it feel to be walking a mile a day?" This language leads them into the concept of future vision without abruptly saying "Let's set a goal to. . . ."
2. Goals should have a recognizable timeline or story. In other words, consider including progress status associated with the goal. Some programs use percentage; others use readiness to change language.
3. Goals should also have a status of met, not met, and perhaps not applicable. This allows for easy viewing of active goals and final resolution of completed goals.
4. Goal language should always be in the first person and have a time element to it: "I will learn to monitor my blood glucose by November 12."
5. Goal language should be clear and provide enough detail for goals to be understood well after they are written.
6. Keep the goal realistic. Keeping the goal small enough to be accomplished in a short time provides a sense of progress for all concerned.
7. Try not to have too many goals at a time. Two to four goals are about as many as anyone can handle at one time. Some people can only handle one.

This chapter sets forth general components of a disease management program. There are programs that have all, some, or more of these components. The key is to understand where the disease manager fits in the scheme of the program design and be a willing and capable participant in the design when called to do so.

CHALLENGE QUESTIONS

1. What is the most critical aspect of a disease management program?
2. Should disease managers be deeply involved in the design of the program?
3. Should a disease manager take advantage of educational opportunities while completing an assessment?

CHAPTER 9

Operational Considerations for Disease Managers

OVERVIEW

How disease managers practice is a genuine challenge. This chapter provides an overview of the operational elements necessary to provide a successful service. The content primarily applies to disease managers who practice in groups such as a department or call center.

Quite often, disease managers find themselves within a program design that has clinical and operational expectations. An example of a clinical expectation is that the disease manager will capture all medication names, dosing, and instructions for each patient. Another clinical expectation is that all heart failure patients not on an ACE inhibitor will be prompted to speak to their physician about taking one. The clinical expectations are by far the easiest segment of the disease manager's role.

Operational expectations in a call center are almost always foreign to disease managers because they typically have not had exposure to a call center environment, so they do not have a reference point. An example of an operational expectation is that the disease manager will maintain a contact rate of at least four patients per hour or that they will have less than 5 percent of their newly contacted members opt out of the program. These metrics sound more like assembly-line work and are difficult to embrace.

The following sections will shed light on the how and why behind disease management operations.

PRIMARY DISEASE MANAGEMENT MODEL

One of the first issues to understand is how the disease manager relates to his or her patients. In the primary disease management model, one person is assigned to one disease manager. The primary model is normally reserved for higher acuity situations where the need is intense and continuity of care is paramount. Disease managers naturally prefer the primary model because the relationship developed over the interactions is pleasing to both parties.

Some argue that the primary model is necessary for sound behavior change. They will tell you that the trust and credibility that builds over time is the secret to an efficient and effective relationship. Nursing departments have struggled with this for years. In the early years, primary nursing was the norm. A patient had his or her own nurse. When the hospital census was up and the number of available nurses was down, the primary nursing requirement was not attainable. The same thing happens in disease management because disease management is a volume business; the more patients contacted, the greater the impact.

From a purely cost-of-delivery perspective, the primary model is more expensive to deliver and is not as efficient as the team model. In fact, operational statistical methodologies demonstrate that the primary care model is four to six times more expensive that the team model. The cost of delivery in the primary disease management is justified when the savings opportunity of the population served covers the cost. Refer back to the discussion of value proposition in Chapter 4 for a review of how this might be true.

Clearly, the primary disease management model works well in the right situations, but there are drawbacks. Scheduling can become an issue because the disease manager–patient interaction is highly dependent in them being at the same place at one time. Also, because there is a one-nurse–to–one-patient relationship, if there isn't an opportunity to learn from a variety of disease managers who may have different areas of expertise.

TEAM DISEASE MANAGEMENT MODEL

The team disease management model, one disease manager assigned to many patients, is the usual operational model for many reasons. First, few cost models will support the cost of a primary disease manager. Second, experience tells us that there is not a significant difference between the effectiveness of the two models for the less acute person. Finally, the team will not likely be ill, go on vacation, or be in a meeting at the same time, thus leading to a much greater likelihood of contacting or being available for the patient.

No right answer exists to how many disease managers to have on a team. If maximum efficiency is more important than ensuring the patient has a chance of speaking to the same person at least every third time, then as many as 12 to 20 disease managers can work together. If there is a strong desire to keep the team as small as possible while still enjoying some efficiency, then the team can be as small as three to five.

PROGRAM PARTICIPATION STRATEGIES

Enrollment and engagement are the two ways a patient can join and participate in a disease management program. Both are viewed as voluntary. The enrollment method requires a patient to enroll in the program in order to participate. The patient opts in to the program when asked. The patient roster grows as patients agree to join.

The engagement method assumes that all patients are participants until they request to leave the program; the patient opts out of the program. The patient roster decreases as patients opt out.

Disease manager roles differ in the enrollment and engagement models. Table 9.1 highlights the role expectations.

Table 9.1 Disease Manager Role Expectations per Program Participation Method

Disease Manager Expectations	Enrollment	Engagement
Tone of first contact	Sell program and close deal. Perhaps use scripting to ensure key selling points are mentioned.	Instruct patient on disease management benefit. Convince patient of the value of the program they are already in.
Patient roster	Add patient to group.	Keep patient in group.
Value proposition	Tends to focus on only patients in the program.	Based upon entire identified population even though some may opt out.
Measuring value	Measure only patients who are continuously enrolled.	Measure entire group regardless of contact.

LENGTH OF THE CALL

The length of call per patient has always been a subject of great debate. Call times can range from a few minutes to more than an hour. On average, most disease managers spend between 15 to 20 minutes with each patient. Table 9.2 demonstrates a typical encounter timeline.

This table points to the reality of a disease manager's central challenge: to affect the patient's health status in a relatively short amount of time. Refer to the call time breakdown in Table 9.3 and Figure 9.1 to see a breakdown of what an average patient will receive in any given year.

One can readily determine that the disease manager must make good use of the time given them. According to this example, 20 percent of the time is spent on entering and leaving the conversation, 30 percent of the time is spent confirming administrative and medication information, and the remaining 50 percent of the time completing an assessment and reviewing care plan elements, such as goals and educational topics.

The operational model should allow for the disease manager to allot more or less time to each category based on patient need. There are some patients who only need a 5 to 10 minute call every now and then to keep them on track. Others are much more needy and will require hour-long phone calls. The point is that this averages out over the course of the calls.

Table 9.2   Encounter Time Line

Call Minute	Activity	Total Minutes
0–2	Introduction; pleasantries	2
3–5	Confirm physician; check on current health status	3
6–8	Confirm current medications; add, edit, or delete medications if necessary	3
9–13	Complete an assessment	5
14–18	Set or review treatment goals; educate; listen to challenges	5
19–20	Schedule next call; warm goodbye	2

Table 9.3   Call Breakdown

Call Breakdown	Call 1	Call 2	Call 3	Call 4	Call 5	Total
Introduction; pleasantries	2	2	2	2	2	**10**
Confirm physician; check on current health status	3	3	3	3	3	**15**
Confirm current medications; add, edit, or delete medications if necessary	3	3	3	3	3	**15**
Complete an assessment	5	5	5	5	5	**25**
Set or review treatment goals; educate; listen to challenges	5	5	5	5	5	**25**
Schedule next call; goodbye	2	2	2	2	2	**10**
Total call time	**20**	**20**	**20**	**20**	**20**	**100**

Figure 9.1   Total Call Time per Year

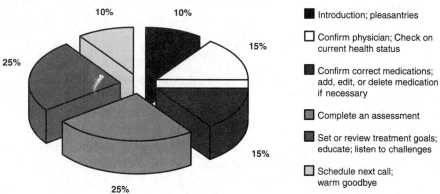

10%   10%   15%   25%   25%   15%

- ■ Introduction; pleasantries
- □ Confirm physician; Check on current health status
- ▨ Confirm correct medications; add, edit, or delete medication if necessary
- ▦ Complete an assessment
- ■ Set or review treatment goals; educate; listen to challenges
- ▢ Schedule next call; warm goodbye

GUIDING THE CONVERSATION

The disease manager must also be a master in guiding a conversation in a manner that does not appear pushy or rude. For patients who are verbose, this is a real challenge. One potential cause of the verbosity is that the patient is not articulate by nature and so will use more words than necessary. The seasoned disease manager realizes that they must be on a pace throughout the day in order to contact the patients on the list. Because of this, every effort must be made to keep the conversation focused.

There are tried-and-true ways to keep the conversation on topic:

1. Introduce each section of the phone call giving an expectation of what should occur.
    a. "Mr. Jones, I would like to ask you about your medications. Please read each of the labels to me one at a time. I'll ask more about them when we are finished with the list."
    b. "Mr. Jones, I have 12 questions to ask you about your heart problem. Please listen for the best answer and say it back to me. Your first response is probably the best. We will go over the results of the assessment when we are done. Are you ready?"
2. Allow the patient to speak until they tire out at the beginning of the call. Most patients cannot talk uninterrupted for more than 2 minutes. Doing this creates an illusion that you are a listener, their point is well heard, and this will put them at ease for the rest of the call.
3. Be in the habit of gentle interruption. Do not be silent for more than 30 seconds. Make liberal use of small comments when they talk such as, "OK," "That's good," "Is that so?", and "Right." Doing this will give you a natural entry into the conversation if it strays too far off course.
4. Let the patient know where they are in relationship to the entire call. Say, "We are about halfway done; let's spend a few minutes talking about your blood glucose monitoring."
5. Reward efficient patients. Praise them for their ability to stay on the topic and cooperate. Tell them that this helps the process, and they will get more from the phone call.

There are also patients who will not or are unable to express themselves well. This kind of patient is not that common, but can be unsettling to the disease manager because this feels like the conversation is unfriendly and strained. There is no best way to approach this situation, but there are things that can be done to validate the tone of the call so that both parties are comfortable with each other. First, make a gentle observation that the patient seems to be quiet or is using few words. Making this observation right away will allow the patient to say that they are troubled, are that way all the time, or that they are not pleased that someone is calling them about their health status.

Second, encourage the patient to elaborate when necessary. Use phrases like, "And then what?" or "What about the pain?" Most patients will open up over time when they gain in comfort and trust.

ANCILLARY STAFFING

Many disease managers have support from persons such as licensed practical nurses, medical technicians, and administrative assistants, who do not engage in the actual act of disease management. For the most part, this staff handles the research and other administrative tasks that surround disease management. Some programs are designed in a way that allows them to conduct certain assessments, make check-in phone calls, and handle in-bound phone calls. Other duties include sending mail, sending and receiving faxes, and scheduling the next phone call with the patient.

DEMAND MANAGEMENT

Demand management refers to responding to a patient's "demand" for answers to a certain clinical situation. In this scenario, patients make a call to the disease manager with a question or situation. More than 90 percent of the time, the patient has a symptom that is bothersome enough to ask someone else; they need on-demand, expert help. This presents an interesting challenge for a disease management program that specializes in one or two conditions because the subject of the call may not be related at all to the specialty of the program. Demand management can take three major types: clinical judgment, guideline, or algorithms.

Clinical Judgment

The clinical judgment refers to the process of taking the patient's question and responding based on the expertise and experience of the disease manager. In this case, they do not rely on reference material to provide answers. The disease manager records the call in narrative or SOAP-note format. Here is an example result of a demand management call in SOAP-note format:

Subjective: 69-year-old diabetic patient has had multiple episodes of late morning lightheadedness and hunger over the last 3 weeks. Denies shortness of breath, chest pain, fainting, slurred speech, or confusion.

Has not changed medications nor changed how they take them. No prior history of similar events. Recently started mall walking.

Objective: Patient's home blood glucose reading during one of these events was 68mg/dl.

Assessment: Probably hypoglycemic reaction.

Plan: Continue to monitor blood glucose during the events; instructed to speak to doctor about adjusting insulin dosing now that activity pattern has changed; taught hypoglycemic reversal technique; call back to us if there are more questions.

Guidelines

The second demand management type is guidelines. Guidelines are a list of symptoms and signs that are usually categorized by urgency. The guidelines are separated by topics such as "pediatric with fever" or "adult chest pain." The disease manager will probe for elements in each category to determine the necessary action. Categories are normally based on location such as self-care (home), clinic appointment, or emergency room.

The guideline may contain simple logic that steers the disease manager to choose one category over the other. For instance, a rule may be that any checkmark in the emergency room category means that the person should head for the emergency room. In another method, there may be a requirement to have at least three checkmarks in a column to make a decision.

For guidelines, the disease manager simply checks the appropriate elements and records the disposition of the call.

Algorithms

The most precise and accurate decision-making demand management type is the algorithm. In this type, the disease manager follows a predefined set of questions that have yes or no answers. The response to the question leads to the next logical question. Like guidelines, the algorithms have titles. It is up to the disease manager to select the correct title to begin the questioning. Algorithms can be paper or automated. In either form, the more sophisticated variety also allows for skipping to another algorithm if necessary.

Any algorithm has end points: places that draw a final conclusion about the situation. The end points generally refer to the same categories as the guidelines, but because they are more diagnostically precise, may be more specific. A well-written algorithm can suggest a doctors appointment in 6 hours, 12 hours, or in 2 weeks, for instance. Some automated algorithms have way points that represent points of interest on the way to the final conclusion. A way point is like a thought one has in the middle of investigation that should not be forgotten and should be addressed along with the final conclusion. The clinical judgment example illustrates this point through the mention of the lack of regular blood glucose monitoring during a symptomatic event. This was a point that should be registered and then brought up later for reconciliation.

Recording the results of a manually completed algorithm may be as simple as documenting the title of the algorithm and the conclusion. Automated versions record the entire path taken through the algorithm.

CASE MANAGEMENT INTERACTION

Disease managers often interact with case managers. Usually, the direction of communication is disease manager to case manager; it is rarely the other way around. Disease managers refer patients based on a prearranged list of conditions or situations that are potential case management cases.

The key to a successful interaction between these closely related professions is in the understanding of the underlying purposes of the roles. Because case managers are largely in a reactive mode responding to catastrophic events or hospitalizations, they are in a mode of resource and service needs. This is not a core attribute of disease management. Toward this end, communications should be limited to requests for benefit explanations, resource coordination, or transfer to a more intensive case management environment for a short while.

Likewise, case managers who have access to patients who are in a clinical decompensation trajectory, but who do not require the noted services, should consider referring their patients to the disease manager.

PHYSICIAN INTERACTION

The degree of physician interaction varies greatly across disease management programs. The intensity of physician interaction is dictated by the disease management setting. If the program is colocated or directly affiliated with physician practices, then the communication can be much more intense than a health plan–sponsored telephonic model.

Disease management program designers spend a great deal of time crafting physician interventions. This is because of the two-way importance of trying to support or not interfere with physician practices. For the most part, physicians are not compensated for or are expecting to support the overhead for disease management programs. Something as simple as a clinical status report from a disease manager can be more of a disruption to the physician despite best intentions because it needs to be reviewed, filed in a chart, and potentially acted upon.

Whatever the degree of physician interaction, disease managers should always consider themselves in a supporting role to the physician-patient relationship. In some ways, the disease manager provides services between clinic visits. In this capacity, the patient comes to know and understand best practices and has a forum for questions, clarifications, and problem solving.

Over the years, disease managers have learned to not overload the physician with contact. The most appreciated action is a redirection back to the physician's office in the case of an emerging troubling symptom. Back to the value proposition for disease management, this prevents an unnecessary emergency room visit or hospitalization.

CHALLENGE QUESTIONS

1. What are the challenges with the team disease manager model?
2. Why is disease management so effective when, according to the example given in this chapter, the average patient requires 100 minutes a year on the phone?
3. What are the best ways to handle the physician contact issue?

CHAPTER 10

Patient Counseling Techniques

————— **OBJECTIVES** —————

1. Describe the major tenets of shared and informed decision making.
2. Define the principles of goal setting.

OVERVIEW

Disease managers use a variety of counseling methods to assist their patients to improve their health status. Training in this area is usually weak in nursing, dietician, and pharmacist specialties. Health educators and exercise physiologists have slightly more. This chapter will explore the shared decision-making and goal-setting counseling techniques.

PATIENT COUNSELING IN DISEASE MANAGEMENT

Before diving into these techniques, it is helpful to put patient counseling into the context of disease management practice. Because disease management is designed to improve health status, one must understand individual health characteristics, identify issues that will prevent or worsen health, and then provide guidance to improve those issues. Providing guidance can take several forms, from declarative statements, "Make an appointment to have your blood pressure checked," to information sharing, "Let me tell you about why blood pressure control is necessary," to discussion format, "What do you think about your blood pressure control?" Because disease management programs depend on the persuasiveness of the disease manager to cause the patient to act, all three approaches are used to some extent.

The disease manager must take care to apply the right approach to the right situation at the right time. Using declarative statements for all health issues will not work, for instance. Also, be careful not to create an atmosphere of teacher and pupil when it is not appropriate. Younger patients may be resistant to lectures; older persons may want to be told what to do and not want to understand the entire issue before acting.

Here is a general scheme for using the most effective approach:

Declarative approach: Use the declarative approach when there is a solid trust and credibility base in the interaction. The declarative approach uses simple, yet bold, statements such as, "You should lose 15 pounds over the next three months." This statement is made with the full expectation of the weight loss without need for explanation. When trust is there, and the request is reasonable, this approach works quite well.

Information sharing: Use the information-sharing approach when the patient asks for more information. Telling a patient something when they are not asking for it is not effective. Unfortunately, disease managers do this all the time out of habit. They develop scripts for health topics and will go on regardless of the patient's desire to know. As was covered in Chapter 11, a patient must be motivated to extend their knowledge before they learn, and knowledge and behavior are sometimes unrelated.

Discussion format: Use the discussion format to ease into the subject of the conversation; to get the patient to act or behave in a certain way. Keep the discussion focused on the topic at hand and keep the conversation short. A patient will express their tendency to want to know or be told what to do rather quickly.

INFORMED AND SHARED DECISION MAKING

Informed and shared decision making is a popular method used by disease managers to help a person arrive at a conclusion about a health issue. The U.S. Preventive Services Task Force (USPSTF), in collaboration with the Task Force on Community Preventive Services, defines informed decision making (IDM) as an individual's overall process of gathering relevant health information from both his or her clinician and from other clinical and nonclinical sources, with or without independent clarification of values.[1] The task force defines shared decision making (SDM) as a particular process of decision making by the patient and clinician in which the patient:

1. Understands the risk or seriousness of the disease or condition to be prevented.
2. Understands the preventive service, including the risks, benefits, alternatives, and uncertainties.

3. Has weighed his or her values regarding the potential benefits and harms associated with the service.
4. Has engaged in decision making at a level at which he or she desires and feels comfortable.[2]

The techniques used for SDM are not universal. Some techniques require a full disclosure of all benefits and risks (taken from the legacy informed consent); some emphasize the collaborative nature of arriving at a decision where the clinician does not state a preference; and others require the clinician to let their preference be known.

SDM is a process that, in theory, seems to be a perfect match for disease management practice. This may not be true in all circumstances. SDM has positive and negative attributes worthy of consideration.

The negative points include:

1. SDM takes time. The process requires skillful interaction between the parties that, in turn, requires time. For many disease management initiatives, this is not a scalable solution.
2. SDM mandates enough knowledge on the disease manager's behalf to understand treatment alternatives along with their risks and benefits. Although common issues, such as whether to get an angiogram or participate in a smoking cessation class, are relatively easy to know, the list of issues is endless and no one disease manager can know enough to help guide the decision.
3. SDM is not for everybody. Some people want to be told what to do, and some people cannot be told what to do. Determining which one you are talking to is difficult in the time allotted to each patient.
4. SDM requires patients to understand medicine. They must learn that medicine does not have all the answers; that there is an art and a science to treatments; that opinions vary across treatment providers; that some treatments are investigational; and that learning the strength of evidence affects recommendations.
5. SDM requires that patients have a base knowledge to absorb the relatively complicated medical terminology and concepts.

The positive points include:

1. SDM, when done correctly, ensures that a patient is in full understanding of what they are about to do and may improve clinical outcomes because of that.
2. SDM at the point of service is an effective counseling tool for those who are facing tough treatment choices.
3. SDM offers an alternative to traditional or parent-child medical relationships.

Disease managers should not shy away from using SDM because it appears that there are more negative than positive points. It is this way because this counseling mechanism is not well studied, and there is much more to be learned. Here are a few instances where SDM may fit:

Should I go to the doctor to ask about an insulin pump?

What are the treatment options for having a gallstone removed?

Should I get a flu shot?

When do I consider seeing a specialist for my heart problem?

GOAL SETTING

Goal setting is another common counseling method used by disease managers. Goal setting as a technique to accomplish tasks is not unique to health care and is a tried-and-true method for those who respond to the notion of attaining a goal.

Who wants to set goals? That is a good question because goal setting is not really a common behavior, and it may not always be the time to set a goal. First, there are very few people who have the discipline to think of, then write down (in measurable wording), personal or professional goals. Most persons are not in the habit of promising to commit a future act, although it may be more popular among the educated, where goal attainment is a hallmark of success. For the people who are not inclined, the concept can be foreign. When the disease manager says, "Would you like to set a goal to walk 2 miles everyday?" the patient may or may not understand the meaning of that phrase.

Second, setting a goal implies that the person is ready to set a goal. Let's say that a disease manager asks a smoker to set a goal to choose a smoking cessation method in the next week. If the person has not decided to quit smoking, the conversation should be centered on informed or shared decision-making techniques instead. Once the person has decided to take action, goal setting can begin.

Goals challenge the patient to succeed, to move in a particular direction, and to claim victory once there. Goals may be accomplished with or without knowledge of the reason behind the goal. Few diabetics can comprehend the meaning of a microalbumin lab test, but they can and do set goals to get one. The disease manager may use the counseling techniques mentioned in this chapter or others to convince the patient to set a goal. As was stated earlier, there are some patients who will not commit to a goal. Do not be discouraged by this. Instead, find an alternative mechanism that they are comfortable trying, such as a simple checklist.

Goals are created in context of an issue. The best way to think of a goal is that it rests in the middle of an issue and one or more tasks. Let's look at the following schema:

Issue
   Goal(s)
      Tasks(s)

Let's take an example of how this would work using multiple goals.

Issue: Patient smokes
   Goal: Convince patient that smoking is harmful
      Task: Call patient and mention harmful effects of smoking
   Goal: Agree to stop smoking
   Goal: Have a plan for smoking cessation
      Task: Choose quit method
      Task: Choose date
      Task: Quit smoking on the chosen date

In this example, goals are part of a larger issue. Some goals need more detail, and that is when tasks come in handy. Instead of tasks, patients may call these reminders.

Crafting a goal is fairly easy once the parameters are well understood. Standard goal writing follows the SMART format. A goal must be:

- **S**pecific
- **M**easurable
- **A**ttainable
- **R**ealistic
- **T**angible with a target date

Ideally, goals should be written from the patient's perspective. Some goals are not patient goals, and they should be written from the eyes of the writer. Examples of well-written patient goals are:

1. I will be able to walk to the end of my driveway without assistance by next Friday.
2. I will have a complete medication list when I see my doctor next month.
3. I will be able to explain what to do when my blood sugar gets too low when I speak to my daughter this afternoon.

Goals should have a status of met or not met. Progress toward the goal can be expressed in a variety of ways. Most disease managers prefer to create a running narrative of the progress toward the goal.

RESOURCES

The following resources represent a solid cross-section of goal setting and shared/informed decision-making information.

- Paula Jorde Bloom. *Circle of Influence: Implementing Shared Decision Making and Participative Management (Director's Toolbox)*. New Horizons, January 2000.
- Dennis J. Mazur. *Shared Decision Making in the Patient-Physician Relationship: Challenges Facing Patients, Physicians, and Medical Institutions*. Tampa, FL: American College of Physician Executives, 2001.
- Gary Ryan Blair. *Goal Setting 101: How to Set and Achieve a Goal!* The GOALSGUY, 2000.
- Anna Juarez. *The Setting Goals and Achieving Them Method*. Work Book, Self-Published, 2002. ISBN 0971446318.

CHALLENGE QUESTIONS

1. Is goal setting too narrow an approach? It seems as if goals can be too small.
2. How many goals can a person handle at a time?
3. How does a goal relate to the value proposition of the disease management program?
4. Is shared decision making too costly? How does shared decision making relate to goal setting?

Endnotes

1. Briss, P., Rimer, B., Reilly, B., et al. "Promoting Informed Decisions About Cancer Screening in Communities and Healthcare Systems." *American Journal of Preventive Medicine* 26, no. 1 (2004):67–80.

2. U.S. Preventive Services Task Force. *Guide technical preventive services report of the U.S. Preventive Services Task Force, 2nd ed.* Washington, DC: Office of Disease Prevention and Health Promotion, U.S. Government Printing Office, 1996.

CHAPTER 11

Behavior Change

OBJECTIVES

1. Define the difference between behavior change and adherence.
2. List at least three foundational behavior theories and their primary intent.
3. List three health-related behavior change theories and provide a short explanation of each.
4. Describe at least seven techniques disease managers can use to enhance the likelihood of behavior change.

OVERVIEW

The effectiveness of any disease management program depends upon the degree to which behavior change occurs in the target population. In this sense, behavior change belongs to patients, physicians, health plans, and even government agencies. For the purposes of this chapter, behavior change is defined as sustained difference in habit, attitude, or intention. Affecting true behavior change is certainly the holy grail for disease managers, and like any holy grail, it is difficult to find.

CHANGING BEHAVIOR

Behavior change is at both the individual and population level. For the individual, behavior change includes removing barriers, motivational interventions, encouraging positive attitudes, teaching coping strategies, and problem solving. At the population level, behavior change includes awareness campaigns, providing access to care or information, and ensuring the infrastructure for optimal care delivery.

Behaviors can be simple to complex; behaviors can be health promoting or health demoting. In order to gain a common understanding, let's review a few scenarios that disease managers will encounter in the chronically ill population.

Eating—eat too much, eat the wrong thing, eat too fast, eat too much when stressed, eat too much when happy

Exercise—does not prefer taxing the body, does not do anything that intentionally raises the heart rate

Tobacco—uses tobacco, uses tobacco around children or other nonsmokers, exposes themselves to environmental tobacco smoke

Alcohol—consumes more than two alcohol drinks per day, drinks and drives, becomes angry or violent when drinking

Medication—forgets to take medications, takes too many medications

Self-management—does not regularly monitor their blood glucose, weight, peak flow

Medical care—will not make or keep medical appointments, is passive during medical appointments, will not follow care plan instructions

Sleep—does not get adequate sleep

Stress—overly anxious reaction to events

These behaviors are observable and thus can be measured. What lies underneath the causation of the behavior remains a mystery. What prompts a person to behave in a certain way? Theologians will say that behavior is a function of free will. That is probably the best explanation, but the most frustrating to those who are trying to affect behavior change.

Even though it seems almost impossible to change another's behavior, it is not. There are guiding principles and techniques that have been shown to work at some level, and many can be employed by disease managers. The remainder of this chapter describes these methods in some detail and applies the methods to disease management practice.

BEHAVIOR CHANGE FOR DISEASE MANAGERS

First things first. For disease managers, behavior change starts at home and their own behaviors can affect their effectiveness. Disease managers who smoke, for instance, are prone to avoid or minimize smoking cessation interventions. Disease managers are people too. They have their own approaches to life and health that may be in direct opposition to the daily messages to be as healthy as possible. The most effective disease managers have gone through a reconciliation process in which they have carefully examined their own habits and attitudes, understand how that has affected their approach, and made appropriate adjustments. This may mean that they alter their own behaviors to be consistent with their message or have made a conscious decision to help others who can't or won't help themselves in certain ways. Sometimes the teacher learns the most. Because of the sensitivity of the issue, the begin-at-home approach to behavior change is rarely addressed in an overt way.

BEHAVIOR CHANGE: PAST TO PRESENT

Behavior change principles and understanding have been in a constant state of evolution. The common themes across all of the behavior change theories are life experience, motivation, and human response. Behavior change theories are also closely associated with learning, absorbing, and then doing or behaving in a particular way. Disease managers use this paradigm all the time. The difficulty comes in drawing clear causation between the intervention and the resultant behavior.

Unfortunately, behavior change instruction is limited in the basic professional training of who becomes a disease manager. Behavior change theory is taught as a part of the orientation of a larger course of instruction and perhaps reinforced at regular intervals. It will help to understand how behavior change principles have formed by reviewing the timeline. The following principles have had staying power.

Experience is the best teacher.

"If you tell me, I will listen. If you show me, I will see. But if you let me experience, I will learn." The 5th-century B.C. philosopher Lao-Tse developed what we now call a case study using a beginning scenario in the form of a parable. The group then discusses and explores all possibilities.

Using questioning as a means to learn.

In 300 B.C., Socrates, and later his student, Plato, would teach students by asking questions. His premise was that the "teacher" was not the expert, but instead would guide the discussion through a series of questions which the learner would attempt to answer. This process is a form of self-generated understanding; the gentle laying out of knowledge and intentions for the learner to realize what was important. For many years, this was considered to be the best way of learning and is often used today in the form of challenge-based learning. A scenario is placed before the learner, then a series of questions are put before them to expose gaps in reasoning and obtain new knowledge.

Aristotle (384–322 B.C.) added the notion of ensuring a well-balanced environment that included science, physical training, debate, and philosophy. He also thought that learning occurs through life, and that the learner has different emphases throughout life. Aristotle pioneered the concept that people learn through association between ideas, promoted recall, and sustained behavior as a result of that knowledge. John Stuart Mill (1806–1873), a later theorist, added to this by challenging that all behavior is affected by simple ideals. He thought a behavior was far more complex because the resultant behavior resembles the original component ideas.

During the early to mid-1800's, systematic learning took hold; this is what we call a lesson plan or curriculum today. The thought was that systematic learning was a way to ensure a progression from novice to expert. Interestingly, this was called technology, from the Greek word *techne*—referring to art, craft, or skill.

Behavior can be learned.

Behaviorism came from the educational research of Ivan Pavlov and Vladimir Mikhailovich Bekhterev, two Russian psychologists. In their well-known research, they were able to demonstrate that if you made a sound while feeding a dog, then after some repetition, when the food was replaced with only the sound, the dog would still salivate. This is known as classical conditioning and is used today in many forms. Disease managers use this method when they teach that when the blood glucose monitor readings are in the normal range, the patient should feel better about their self-control and be motivated to keep the momentum going by eating correctly and exercising.

John B. Watson added to this idea by suggesting that behavior is a function of habit. Habits are formed by repetition and recency. For instance, early training may teach a boy to allow girls to go through the door first. A lifetime of this habit becomes automatic due to the frequency and constancy of this behavior. Disease managers hope to instill better health habits by encouraging patients to have habits like placing their pills in the pill box on Sunday night or weighing themselves every morning.

Memorizing versus understanding.

The founder of gestalt psychology, Max Wertheimer (1880–1943), found that persons who learned through memorization were unable to use the information in any other way than the context in which it was learned. Memorization was learned under rigid rules, thus limiting association with other facts. Learners who were taught the underlying principles could easily generalize knowledge to other situations and thus participate in critical thinking.

Behavior is a result of motivation to reach a higher need.

Abraham Maslow's hierarchy of needs is a well-known model to the health care professional and probably is still in the memory of most disease managers. In Maslow's model, behavior is geared to assure lower needs, such as the need for safety. Once a level is attained, higher levels, such as food, are addressed. Maslow was a humanist who shied away from the classical scientific model. He believed that behavior change is also affected by experiences over time. As an example, a young parent will have a generally different reaction to an issue than an older parent.

Disease managers who interact with adolescent diabetics will tell you that even though the younger diabetics have the same therapies to control their diabetes, they are managed quite differently from the self-care perspective.

Practice makes perfect.

Edwin Guthrie theorized that skills could be broken up into acts, which are then made up of movements. Movements require physical activity of some sort and are in response to specific stimuli. All these parts require practice to draw associations for skill acquisition; the more practiced, the more skillful. How does this apply to disease management? There are physical skills associated with the common chronic diseases: insulin drawing and injecting, blood glucose monitoring, and peak flow meter reading are a few examples. All of these are technique dependent and the more skillful the patient, the better the outcome.

If we practice long enough, then visual imagery is possible. Picture the downhill skier about to start a slalom race. They visually cover the course gate by gate before starting the race. This speaks to giving the patient enough time to master skills.[1]

Concentrated practicing is not as effective as practice that incorporates rest periods or adequate time before the next practice session.[2] The lesson for disease managers is to allow the patient to practice simple tasks over a several-day period. This will ensure a higher level ability to perform the skill. Think of a newly diagnosed insulin requiring diabetic. Traditionally they get 5 minutes with an orange practicing injection before they are asked to inject themselves. Spreading this out over several days will build skill level and confidence.

You behave that way because of who you are and where you are.

Kurt Lewin, a renowned social scientist of the 1940s and 1950s, developed the field theory that postulates that behavior is a function of the person and their environment. This is translated to personal attributes and the social context drives behavior.

Lewin's work also demonstrated that learning occurs when there is a conflict between what the person knows at the moment of learning and the abstract notion of the new behavior. This conflict breeds a cycle of action, generalization, and testing. As an example, patients who are currently not exercising and learn that they can look better and feel better by doing a certain round of exercises start by imagining the difference between how they look now and how they could look. This difference spurs them to action, perhaps trying the exercise, making a generalization that if they keep exercising they will reach their mental image of themselves in their new body. They will continue to test this notion by looking in the mirror and weighing themselves.

HEALTH-RELATED BEHAVIOR CHANGE

All of the preceding work provides a foundational understanding of general behavior tendencies. The next three behavior change theories are in widespread use today. They are the health-belief model, the stages of change or transtheoretical model, and the consumer-information processing model.

Health-Belief Model

The health-belief model (HBM) was developed using many of the earlier theories to examine health behavior. The tuberculosis screening campaigns of the 1950s were the stimulus for developing the HBM. Public health departments were puzzled when people were not wanting to get chest X-rays to screen for tuberculosis, even though it was deemed safe and would save many from the ravages of tuberculosis. Social learning theorists (Irwin Rosenstock and Howard Becker) partnered with public health officials to determine how to encourage people to get screened. The result was a better understanding of how to motivate people to be screened and how these motivations applied to other health-related behaviors. The going-in assumption of the theorists was that people feared the disease and possibly the screening test itself and did not feel that the risk was worth the reward.

The HBM can be broken into four constructs: (1) perceived susceptibility, a person's opinion of the chances of getting a certain condition; (2) perceived severity, a person's opinion of how serious this condition is; (3) perceived benefits, a person's opinion of the effectiveness of some advised action to reduce the risk or seriousness of the impact; and (4) perceived barriers, a person's opinion of the concrete and psychological costs of this advised action. Later on, cues to action and self-efficacy were added to the model. Cues to action are those events that stimulate the health-promoting action, such as written materials or a motivational speech. Self-efficacy speaks to the confidence the person has in doing the health action successfully.

The primary usefulness of the HBM is in determining underlying reasons why the person is behaving the way they are, then crafting messages that resonate with that individual. In the example where the person has low self-efficacy and low perceived benefit about starting an exercise program, messages and specific instruction can be tailored to focus on those two aspects.

The health-belief model has two primary limitations. First, the model may be in conflict with nonhealth beliefs and does not provide strategies for accommodating for the conflict. Second, there are times when behavior precedes belief, rendering the HBM less useful as a cause-and-effect model. Nonetheless, the HBM consists of valuable constructs to consider when determining potential underlying causes for a person's health behavior and when used in context of other factors remains a powerful model.

Stages of Change or Transtheoretical Model

James O. Prochaska developed the stages of change model in 1979, and in later work with Carlo DiClemente, refined the model into what it is today. The premise of the stages of change model is that people pass through stages of change while attempting to adopt health-related habits. The original work concentrated on what happens when people attempt to quit smoking, then addictive behaviors. Today, the model is applied to almost any health-related change situation. The stages of change model is otherwise called readiness to change, and describes six stages: (1) precontemplation—the person is unaware of the problem or has not thought seriously about change; (2) contemplation—the person is seriously thinking about a change (in the near future); (3) preparation—the person is planning to take action and is making final adjustments before changing behavior; (4) action—the person implements some specific action plan to overtly modify behavior and surroundings; (5) maintenance—the person continues with desirable actions (repeating the periodic recommended steps while struggling to prevent lapses and relapse); and (6) termination—the person has zero temptation and the ability to resist relapse.

The stages of change model is circular rather than linear. The person may go through several cycles of stages before progressing on to the next. Relapse, the going back to the prior behavior, may send the person back into the first stage. The disease manager finds this model particular useful for describing and tracking the progress of their patients toward making a behavior change. Tactics and messages can be tailored to the present stage.

Consumer-Information Processing Model

The consumer information processing (CIP) model was not developed expressly for health-related behaviors, and although relatively new, has gained widespread adoption in the health care industry. The CIP model provides understanding and strategies for how a person processes health information and is useful for problem solving.

The CIP model distinguishes between knowledge, information, and behavior change. We all have heard the phrase, "Knowledge does not necessarily lead to behavior." In the same manner, information is necessary, but does not necessarily lead to knowledge. According to the model, this can be explained by understanding one's capacity to process information. Literally, this means that a person has an innate and variable capacity to receive, process, and store information.

Adherence

Adherence refers to the durability of the behavior. One can strongly adhere to positive or negative behaviors. Adherence to a health care recommendation is at the heart of disease management outcomes and is a direct result of behavior change initiatives. The adherence literature is replete with discouraging news. As it turns out, adherence is difficult to maintain. Using one representative example of inhaled corticosteroid use in asthmatics, the data challenges the notion that behavior can be changed.

Asthma is a condition that often manifests itself as chest tightness and labored breathing, an uncomfortable and frightening experience. There are well-known and safe treatments to dramatically reduce exacerbations. Despite this fact, many asthmatics do not maintain their treatments. The reasons why this is so puzzles the researchers in a way that is causing a revival of sorts in the way adherence is studied.

Although many adherence strategies have proved ineffective, there are some that show promise:

1. Simple is better. Calling ahead to remind about appointments, leaving reminder notes around the house, and refrigerator magnets have all been shown to have benefit over more elaborate schemes.
2. Accessibility to health information. Readily available information, either in print or verbal, dramatically impacts adherence. People appreciate on-demand expert advice over almost anything else.
3. Monitor adherence. People do better when they know they are watched. This is why home monitoring works in selected situations.
4. Train the health care team adherence strategies. The assumption that the provider's instructions are enough to ensure adherence is not working.
5. Involve more than one person. Adherence works better when the person's family or friends are involved.

DISEASE MANAGER'S ROLE IN BEHAVIOR CHANGE

First and foremost, the disease manager is an agent for behavior change. The information in this chapter describes the dominant constructs used in providing behavior change, but it is still up to the disease manager to discern the need for and institute a plan that incorporates behavior change techniques. The human factor is the wild card in the equation. The following are points that will challenge disease management practice methodology and may lead to more effective behavior change.

1. Listen for cues and underlying reasons behind making or not making changes.
2. Problem solve instead of instruct. Disease management should not be an instructional course.
3. Be positive; encourage whenever possible.
4. Create a feeling of compassionate oversight.
5. Be available.
6. Listen two thirds and talk one third of the time.
7. Always consider situations from the person's orientation. This is known as empathy.
8. Concern yourself with how the messages are delivered. Be concise, clear, and always confirm understanding.
9. Be valuable. Become an expert. Create the "on-demand expert advice" environment.
10. Change methods on the fly. Craft your approach to the person.

CHALLENGE QUESTIONS

1. What aspects of disease management hamper behavior change techniques?
2. Are there techniques disease managers can borrow from other industries? Which industries? Which techniques?

Endnotes

1. Adams, J. "Motor Learning and Retention." In M. Marx and M. Bunch, eds., *Fundamentals and Applications of Learning*. New York: Macmillan, 1977.
2. Hull, C. L. *Principles of Behavior.* Englewood Cliffs, NJ: Prentice Hall, 1943.

CHAPTER 12

Remote Patient Monitoring

———— **OBJECTIVES** ————

1. Define what is meant by remote patient monitoring.
2. Describe the risks and benefits of remote patient monitoring.
3. List the two major classifications of remote devices.
4. Give the operational considerations for ensuring a patient understands how to use the remote device and the purpose of its measurement.

OVERVIEW

Remote patient monitoring has been used for over twenty years, yet its time is just now here. In 1986, the Bayer company introduced the Glucometer M, the first blood glucose meter to contain a memory chip. The Glucometer M effectively obviated the need to maintain a blood glucose log book. A year later, the Bayer company released a personal computer software application that, through the use of a cable that connected the meter to the computer, could capture the meter's data and view it several ways. While this doesn't sound exciting today, it was revolutionary then and would pave the way towards other devices.

Remote patient devices, such as the Glucometer M, represented more than technological progress. They were a means of collecting and analyzing reliable and valid clinical data that was considered more factual than self-recorded data. Today, the devices have advanced to include wrist watches that monitor blood pressure, pulse, and heart rate. The future of remote patient devices is bright, and disease managers will find themselves at the epicenter of the progress and practical use of them.

109

REMOTE PATIENT MONITORING: AN EMERGING TECHNOLOGY

Remote patient monitoring (RPM) is an emerging technology solution used to capture and transmit objective clinical data such as weight, blood pressure, peak flow meter readings, and pulse from patients. This data is stored in clinical information systems and is used in the course of disease management interventions. In some cases, data that is out of range may drive alerts to the disease manager for more timely interaction.

The addition of remotely collected objective data has cracked the problem of self-reported data, but there are other obstacles in the path of true understanding of the final value of this technology. The major obstacles include the understanding of how these RPM devices should be reimbursed, who should use them and for how long, their place in the disease management practice, and the infancy of the technology itself.

Reimbursement for RPM devices remains a struggle. RPM manufacturers are aggressively attempting to loosen Medicare and Medicaid reimbursement as well as managed care benefit structures. Until reimbursement is available for eligible patients, this aspect of disease management practice will not grow substantially.

RPM is primarily used for the highest risk patients because close monitoring is required to determine, and then act upon, a patient who may be decompensating. This is an efficient and effective use of RPM and is the dominant reason why disease management programs have added RPM.

For the disease management programs that use RPM, the technology is both a blessing and a curse. The challenges include identifying the appropriate criteria for patient selection, installing the devices in the patient's home, connecting to existing clinical information systems, policies and procedures for reacting to the streams of data, separating the benefits of the RPM from the rest of the population, and removing the device from the home when it is no longer used. Once these issues are under control, the day-to-day benefits of the remote devices demonstrate clear value because of the richness and timeliness of the data.

The RPM device industry is quite new and so is still determining the best designs for its devices. For the most part, the devices are working, but there are issues around the measurement reliability of the devices, data transmission quality, and durability.

COST OUTCOME RESULTS OF RPM

Not many full-featured research studies exist that demonstrate the value of RPM, but the results of studies in this area are promising. In one study using a weight scale and blood pressure monitoring system, the presence of RPM reduced hospital admission for congestive heart failure (CHF) patients by 95 percent, reduced hospital ER or clinic visits related to CHF by 88 percent, reduced home health visits related to CHF by 83 percent, reduced physician clinic visits by 91 percent, and showed a slower progression in disease status based on the New York Heart Association (NYHA) grade scale through home CHF patient monitoring.[1] Another study using heart failure was able to reduce rehospitalization rate in only 3 months.[2]

REMOTE MONITORING OPTIONS

Disease managers may be exposed to two categories of remote patient monitoring: device and lab. Common devices include those to measure blood pressure, pulse, pulse oximetry, weight, blood glucose, and peak flow. Common home lab tests include Hba1c, cholesterol, HIV, and urine albumin tests. The number and type of both of these categories is increasing rapidly. The Food and Drug Administration (FDA) has a medical device approval program that is currently evaluating hundreds of remote monitoring options.

OPERATIONAL ASPECTS OF RPM

The question is clear from the disease manager's perspective: "How does this fit into my practice?" The answers to this question are an evolving science, but there are at least two major roles for remote monitoring. The first role for remote monitoring is to use objective data as an component of the clinical interaction. The data can be considered as an independent value or as a part of a trend that may influence the disease manager's guidance and sense of urgency. The second purpose is to reinforce a self-care behavior. In this case, the behavior has equal importance to the actual values.

Installing the device requires patient selection rules. The best qualified patients are those who are at continuous risk of decompensating and for which the data might prevent an unnecessary emergency department visit or hospitalization. Patients who have had multiple utilization events in the past year and have advanced disease are the most qualified.

Once installed, the data should be readily available to qualified disease managers. Taking great care to ensure that data does not sit in the system without expert review will be necessary to avoid liability and patient harm issues. The remote device normally comes with separate monitoring software. Rarely does a disease management program staff have the capacity to cleanly integrate the remote device data inside the clinical information system. The presence of an alert value in the monitoring software should be clearly identified. In this way, the disease manager can react appropriately.

User issues are prevalent with remote devices. Quite often the users are elderly, somewhat debilitated persons who are not technologically savvy. They are challenged by the buttons and other mechanical features of the device. They may also not clearly understand what happens to the data they create by using the device. It is not that unusual for a patient to let a family member or friend take their blood glucose or weigh themselves. The disease manager may pick this up in their monitoring systems and act on the erroneous value as if it was real. Too much of this creates an operational slowdown.

The FDA has published the following checklist for patients who have a remote medical device in the home. This checklist should be given to all patients with a device. The patient and disease manager should also document the patient's understanding of the purpose of the device and its use.

As a home care medical device user, you should know how your device works.

Read your patient education information.

Ask your doctor or supplier questions about your device and take notes.

Know what is required to operate your device.

- Check to see if you need electricity, running water, telephone, or computer connections to operate your device.
- Check to see that your home is suited for your device. Will the stairs, doorways, bathrooms, and house wiring present any problems?
- Keep the device's instructions for use close to your device.
- Pay attention to alarms and error messages. Be familiar with what the alarms and error messages mean.
- Follow the instructions as given.
- Call the supplier for help if you do not understand how your device works.
- Report to your doctor or the device supplier any new problems you have with the device.

Take care of your device and operate it according to the manufacturer's directions.

Read your instructions for taking care of your device and follow them for:

- cleaning
- replacing batteries and filters
- protecting your device (e.g. keeping food and drinks away from your device)

- taking the device safely from home to school, work, church, and vacation spots, and checking ahead to see if these other places are suited for your device
- disposing of your medical device according to the manufacturer's instructions

Always have a back-up plan and supplies.

Make sure you know what to do if your device fails.

Have emergency phone numbers for the suppliers, home care agency, doctor, and manufacturer.

- Be sure that you have the after-hour phone numbers for everyone.
- If appropriate, keep extra batteries for your device and know how to replace them.

Educate your family and caregivers about your devices.

Include them in hospital planning meetings or any device demonstrations.

Ask them to do a hands-on demonstration to show they can effectively use the device.

Keep children and pets away from your medical device.

Do not let children play with the dials, settings, on/off switches, tubings, machine vents, or electrical cords.

Do not allow pets to chew or play with the electrical cords.

Check with your supplier to see if you can turn off your device when you are not using it.

Contact your doctor and home health care team often to review your health condition.

Check to see if there are new conditions that may change the way you or your caregiver use the device.

- Are there changes in vision, hearing, or ability to move?
- Have you had an illness, new medicines, or loss of feeling?

Report any serious injuries, deaths, or close calls.

Report these events to the FDA at 1-800-332-1088.

Report these events to your supplier.

The FDA will take action when needed to protect the public's health.

The FDA has highlighted important information for people with a remote device. There are more specific instructions provided with the device, and the disease manager should be familiar with them as well. Some of the reasons why remote devices do not work, or are not used regularly, are due to simple misunderstandings about how the device is used. The following organizations provide helpful information on remote patient devices.

Endorsing organizations

American Association for Home Care: http://www.aahomecare.org

National Association for Home Care: http://www.nahc.org

National Patient Safety Foundation: http://www.npsf.org

Resource organizations

National Family Caregivers Association: http://www.nfcacares.org

Center for Devices and Radiological Health Home Healthcare Committee: http://www.fda.gov/cdrh/cdrhhhc/
(for additional government sources and information)

DEFINITIONS

It is helpful to know that the FDA has official definitions for medical devices versus a home care medical device. These definitions, and other related information, are located on their website—www.fda.gov.

A **medical device** is any product or equipment used to diagnose a disease or other conditions, to cure, to treat, or to prevent disease. The FDA's Center for Devices and Radiological Health regulates medical devices to provide reasonable assurance of their safety and effectiveness.

A **home health care medical device** is any product or equipment used in the home environment by persons who are ill or have disabilities. These persons, or their providers of care, may need education, training, or other health care–related services to use and maintain their devices safely and effectively in their homes or in other places such as work, school, and church. Examples of some home health care devices are ventilators and nebulizers (to help breathing); wheelchairs; infusion pumps; blood glucose meters, apnea monitors, and other home monitoring devices.

CHALLENGE QUESTIONS

1. Are remote devices a liability problem? What measures would you take to limit liability?
2. Which kinds of patients would benefit—or not benefit—from remote monitoring devices?
3. What needs to be in place for better reimbursement policies?
4. Does RPM help avoid unnecessary medical utilization?

Endnotes

1. S.E. Consortium. "Heart Alert," www.heartalert.net/Presentations/SEConsortium_files/frame.htm. Accessed April 25, 2003.
2. Benatar, D. "Outcomes of Chronic Heart Failure." *Archives of Internal Medicine* 163, no. 3 (February 10, 2003):347–352.

Clinical Information Systems

OVERVIEW

Clinical information systems (CIS) are software applications used by disease managers to record the work they do and keep track of the work planned for the future. For the most part, the CIS is developed by the agency delivering the service and so they are not standard in design or sophistication.

The purpose of this chapter is to describe the CIS components, how they may relate to each other, and how the disease manager uses the CIS as a tool. This chapter is not meant to guide CIS design or act as a basis for training because no one CIS will be the same.

BASIC CIS PRINCIPLES

Clinical Information Systems are not all created equal. Some are very sophisticated and powerful, while some are simple data capture tools. The following five principles of data validation, clinical logic, interface, longitudinal design, and reporting separate the sophisticated from the simple system. Large scale operations require that each of these principles are followed closely to ensure operational efficiency and clinical effectiveness.

Data Validation

A comprehensive CIS will have all of the components mentioned in the following section. Each of the components should be designed to capture the data in a reliable and valid way. In the interest of data integrity, the CIS should not allow entry of erroneous data. For example, a CIS user should not be able to say that a person is 150 years old or that someone weighs 3,200 pounds.

Clinical Logic

There is robust debate about how much clinical logic a CIS should contain. Some CIS contain no clinical logic at all, while some may approach full-blown expert systems that present care plans automatically. Given the relatively embryonic state of disease management, far more CIS designs are basic in nature.

Interface

The CIS can be the low point of a disease manager's working environment because the interface forces the disease manager to think like the application rather than the other way around. Unfortunately, CIS developers are not disease managers—and doubly unfortunate, disease managers do not develop a CIS for themselves. The result is often a CIS that thinks and acts like a developer. The disease manager is left to cope with screen designs, data order, and navigation that are not always conducive to efficient and effective disease management.

Longitudinal Design

The CIS should be able to tell a story, follow the patient through time, and demonstrate progress toward a more healthy care pattern. This requires an encounter-based design that displays trends and historical data.

Reporting

Data captured in the CIS should be readily available to all parties in a way that is clear and understandable. The disease manager should have access to their practice patterns, their patients, and key metrics that affect their effectiveness.

CIS COMPONENTS

The following are short descriptions of what each CIS component should be able to do at a minimum:

1. Security
   - Password-protected access.
   - User role allows access to only necessary CIS modules and assigned patients.
2. Schedule/calendar
   - Schedule a day and time in the future.
   - Suggest the number of days to reconnect based on program rules.
   - Display patients to contact by selected date.
   - Display the number of patients contacted.
3. Administrative data
   - Record name, address, and phone number of patient.
   - Record program information.
   - Record other relevant administrative data unique to disease management program.
4. Medications
   - Record medication name, dose, and instructions.
   - Record medication adherence data.
5. Diagnosis
   - Record diagnosis name, onset date, resolved date.
6. Clinical information
   - Present and store assessment, lab, and utilization data.
7. Care plan
   - Enter and display care plan elements with date and progress.
8. Goals
   - Enter and display goals, goal progress, and completion date of each goal.
9. Progress notes
   - Enter a date/time/user stamped note.
   - Display all notes written on the patient.
10. Reference material
    - Store reference material.
    - View and possibly mail reference material to patient.

USING THE CIS

Many disease managers use the CIS while speaking to a patient. Using the CIS while speaking to a patient is not an easy thing for those who have below-average computer skills. Beginning disease managers are even more challenged. The temptation is to write the entire conversation down while speaking to the patient, then enter the information into the CIS after the encounter is over. This is generally due to the CIS not supporting the workflow in a way that is flexible and user friendly. The CIS is supposed to be a tool for data capture, but sometimes the data (conversation) comes in too fast or too scattered to reasonably be entered in the CIS in real time.

Here is a list of ideas for those who would like to improve their skills using the CIS:

1. Write down a usual scenario of your patient encounter. Practice going through the application as if you were in that scenario.
2. Map out the usual navigation on paper, and explain it to someone else. This will help to explain how the pieces go together.
3. Know the content of all drop-down lists in the application—especially the order of the values.
4. If there are assessments, concentrate on the responses and listen for them during your conversation.
5. Learn as many keyboard navigation commands as possible. Most CIS allow the user to use the tab key to move between fields, for instance. Keyboard commands are much faster than using the mouse.
6. Use time spent waiting for the computer to redraw a screen to begin collecting data for the next screen.
7. Know each module by heart. If you find yourself looking for buttons or fields while speaking to a patient, you will be too slow to keep up.
8. If possible, learn how the CIS logic works behind the scenes. Knowing the logic will help you to understand the cause and effect of your actions.
9. If you think you have found an error in the CIS, use the alt-print screen key combination to record what the screen looks like, then use the paste command in your e-mail or word processing application to record it. Also, write down what you were doing when the trouble occurred.

Is It a Bug or Is It an Enhancement?

Strictly speaking, a bug is an error or defect in the programming of the CIS. Usually, a bug is obvious; the application will suddenly stop, go away, or result in an error message that explains the source of the error. Bugs are fixed by developers and usually require a re-installation of the application.

An enhancement is a new design idea that should add value to the CIS. Disease managers are a critically important source of design ideas. Enhancements are expressed in terms of requirements that describe what the CIS should do. Here is a simple example of an enhancement statement: "The system should allow the user to capture medication refill status."

DISEASE MANAGER'S ROLE IN CIS DESIGN

There are times when a disease manager has an opportunity to make suggestions about how the CIS should work. This can be both a welcoming and frightening opportunity. Application design demands a logical approach, but the challenge is that there is no standard workflow.

The developers will ask you what you want and how you want it to work. The best way to respond to this request is to first list the data that should be collected. For example, the data needed for a medication adherence module might be:

Reason for taking medication (text field, 250 characters)

Adherence (choices like excellent, fair, poor)

Issues with medication (none, not effective, too many side effects)

The next step is to say how you want it to work. The easiest way to communicate this is to use what is known as high-level requirements. Here is an example of how this would look using the medication adherence module as an example:

1. The medication adherence module should be accessed from the main medication module.
2. Once in the medication module, the user should have to complete all fields before finishing.
3. Once finished with the medication adherence module, the user should be brought back to the main medication module.

The developers can then use this information to develop a working or clickable prototype that can be reviewed and approved or redone until the prototype satisfies the requirements.

This example is relatively straightforward. A full-fledged CIS is much harder to imagine and communicate to developers. The more exposure to the design and development, the more effective you will be, and the better the CIS will behave when you need it most.

CHALLENGE QUESTIONS

1. Should disease managers be involved in CIS design?
2. What is the difference between a bug and an enhancement?

CHAPTER 14

A Career in Disease Management

———————— **OBJECTIVES** ————————

1. List the variety of common disease management positions.
2. Describe commonalities between the various positions.
3. List the variety of academic preparations necessary to apply for each position.

OVERVIEW

Many exciting opportunities exist for health-related professionals in disease management. For the most part, the opportunities center around call center or telephonic roles, but there are still a fair amount of direct contact roles. The purpose of this chapter is to describe disease management roles that are based on actual job descriptions taken from Web-based job sites.

No reliable industry statistics are available that show how many disease managers are working in the United States. However, the largest concentration of disease managers are employed by disease management service companies. A back-of-the-envelope estimate for the number of disease managers in this group is between 2,500 and 4,000. About 90 percent of these are registered nurses; 10 percent are registered dieticians, pharmacists, respiratory therapists, and health counselors.

Disease managers also work for health insurance companies and hospital systems that have chosen to build their own programs. The professional distribution of disease managers in these settings closely mirrors that of the disease management companies.

The best way to gain a glimpse of the professional opportunities is to review the job postings for disease managers. What follows is a compendium of job postings from an assortment of companies that are looking for a variety of positions. Note common threads such as professional qualifications, health counseling experience, time in profession, and clinical expertise. Also note the commonalities of what the roles/duties contain. Finally, note the vast array of settings, roles, and expectations; there are many ways to be a disease manager! In fact, in a review of just one search engine, there were 940 disease manager positions available at one time.

REGISTERED NURSE

Registered nurses are asked to provide disease management services for persons with coronary artery disease (CAD), congestive heart failure (CHF), diabetes, chronic obstructive pulmonary disease (COPD), asthma, and hypertension. Some programs also open the disease registry to cancer, high-risk pregnancy, rare chronic diseases, hepatitis C, low-back pain, osteoporosis, osteoarthritis, fibromyalgia, acid-related stomach disorders, decubitus ulcer, atrial fibrillation, and urinary incontinence.

Nurses who have all manner of educational preparation are disease managers. Most companies prefer a diverse work knowledge to include emergency room, intensive care, and general medical-surgical experience. Programs that specialize in one or two conditions may require a background in those conditions. For instance, companies with high-risk pregnancy or neonatal programs will hire nurses with these skills.

Nurses are asked to either carry a caseload in primary nursing models or become a member of a team. Nurses are asked to form plans of care that are either proposed by a clinical information system or developed by themselves. These plans of care are always based on well-established guidelines and can be traced back to the predefined program outcomes. Depending on the program, the nurse may be required to have extensive knowledge of several core diseases or know just enough to provide high-level interventions across many conditions. Almost all programs require a general knowledge or provide training in behavior-change techniques, motivational interviewing, and telephonic skills (where appropriate).

The primary duties for nurses are:

- Performs administrative duties to include engaging patients, explaining program details, conducting and scheduling patients, and ensuring that contact information is current.
- Conducts clinical assessments.
- Forms care plans—perhaps across one or many conditions.
- Provides interventions to patients and their families that may include goal setting, care coordination with the primary care provider or case manager, and provision of relevant written material.

- Documents interactions that are helpful for other care team members and are consistent with quality tracking mechanisms.
- Refers appropriate patients to other health team members when the opportunity arises.
- May participate in ongoing training of fellow disease managers.
- May be asked to obtain certifications or specialized training consistent with the disease management program objectives.

Other knowledge, skills, and abilities include:

- Knowledge of managed care and disease management principles, and how these two create value for each other.
- Experience with educating adult learners.
- Able to communicate effectively with health care team members such as physicians, case managers, family members, and others who may be involved with the care of the patient.
- Experience being a member of a health care team.
- Able to participate in quality management programs. Should have a basic understanding of how quality metrics are used for program improvement.
- Experience in telephonic or call centers.
- Skill in multitasking in a high-volume environment.
- Strong computer skills for programs that require the interaction to be tracked with a clinical information system.
- Flexibility to work in a rapidly changing environment.
- Skills outside of the medical environment. Some programs have specific language requirements, especially Spanish.

PHARMACIST

Pharmacists are asked to do many of the same things that their nursing colleagues are asked to do, but with an emphasis on pharmaceutical management. Mainstream, commercial disease management programs are just beginning to hire pharmacists. As of this writing, pharmacists are more likely to be hired by programs that are sponsored by pharmaceutical companies, hospitals, and specialty disease management programs in which medication management is paramount to obtaining the value proposition.

Typically, disease management programs are looking for licensed pharmacists with patient-contact experience, the ability to communicate rather complex medication information to persons in an effective manner, experience with health plan pharmacy-benefit plans, and who have worked in a variety of settings.

The principal responsibilities are similar to registered nurses. Additional duties include:

- Evaluation of medication profiles for appropriateness, potential efficacy gains, polypharmacy, and drug abuse.
- Medication education to include indications, dosing, method of delivery, adverse reactions, and expectation of response to therapy.
- Interaction with physicians when medication reevaluation is necessary.
- Monitoring for response to therapy and alert the health care provider when necessary.
- Interaction with other members of the disease management care team when necessary.

DIETICIAN

Registered dieticians also share many of the primary duties as their registered nurse colleagues. Disease management programs managing conditions that have a strong reliance on proper nutrition such as diabetes, chronic obstructive pulmonary disease, and heart failure hire dieticians. Dieticians are used as in-program consultants and are frequently asked to work with patients who require above-average dietary intervention. Some programs extend the dietician's responsibilities to exercise, smoking cessation, and weight reduction.

Dieticians are expected to have a masters degree, but that is not necessarily required. Additionally, disease management programs prefer to hire dieticians with adult education backgrounds. Because many dieticians have extensive experience with patient education, this requirement is not hard to find. The last requirement is specific experience in evaluating the dietary status of patients with the chronic illnesses most common to the program in which they are seeking employment.

Dieticians are primarily responsible for:

- Dietary assessment appropriate to the condition.
- Evaluation of potential impact of dietary impact on condition.
- Instruction on meal planning, food preparation, and general eating habits, which may extend to family instruction.
- Special dietary instructions for those who are undergoing treatments or procedures that impact eating patterns.
- Basic dietary instruction to other disease manager colleagues.

HEALTH EDUCATOR/HEALTH COUNSELOR

Health educators are generally persons with a degree in health education, exercise physiology, psychology, social work, or occupational health. Disease management programs use health educators for lifestyle-related issues and for general clinical data intake. Examples of these duties include weight management, exercise prescription, smoking cessation, managing stress, finances, social support, and community resources. Some programs are focused on health-risk appraisal or assessment. In this case, the health educator focuses on both health promotion and health risks. There are relatively few commercial disease management companies that perform this service due to market demand, so the opportunity for health educators is somewhat limited. Disease management companies that focus on informed or shared decision making may also use health educators because many of the topics are consistent with the basic educational preparation. Health educators are also less expensive than their colleagues who have nursing, pharmacy, or nutrition degrees. This makes health educators an attractive group to those who are looking to reduce operating expenses.

In general, health educators should have experience with health promotion programs that feature assessment, planning, and teaching. The health educator should also be well versed in adult education principles, behavior modification techniques, and motivational interviewing. When required, the health educator should have specific knowledge and experience with actuarial data related to health risks.

The health educator will be asked to do the following:

- Conduct assessments commensurate with their scope of education.
- Prepare teaching curriculums that focus on a variety of health-related issues.
- Conduct classes and make telephone contact with identified patients.
- Provide general health teaching to their disease management colleagues who may not have the knowledge and experience in certain issues in which they excel.
- Act as a primary health-topic researcher on behalf of their disease manager clinical colleagues. This research may support care planning, teaching, or reading material for one or a group of patients.

FIELD-BASED DISEASE MANAGER

Field-based disease managers are a small but growing version of a disease manager. Their primary purpose is to provide a link between the patient, disease manager, and physician. Toward this end, the field disease managers represent the disease managers making patient contact in the physician's office. The field disease manager will describe program components, communication patterns, and offer assistance in the administration of referring patients into the program, as well as providing physician instructions for patient care back to the disease manager.

Field disease managers are experienced nurses who are able to effectively interact with physicians and their support staff. They are usually well-known in the community and may have worked for many years in the same environments in which they are assigned. The environment may be challenging to break through, so the field disease manager should be prepared to be persistent, positive, and confident that the service they provide is incredibly important to the entire process.

Field disease managers most often work from their homes and cover an assigned region. Sometimes they will be assigned to a large physician group, specialty physician group, or hospital system. When the field disease manager is assigned to the hospital, they may need to pass a certification to interact with their staff.

The duties of a field disease manager include identifying physician offices to target, sorting patients by physician, educating physicians and their staff on the program components, communicating specific standards of care to the physician, and communicating physician instructions back to the disease manager.

POPULATION MANAGER

A population manager is a unique breed of disease manager. The purpose of the population manager is to identify, monitor, track, and provide specific population-based interventions to a group of patients. The population manager role demands a mix of clinical, epidemiological, and operational skills and experience. Few people have this skill mix, often leaving this role in the hands of several support staff, rather than one person.

Another role or responsibility for the population manager is to manage the targeting strategies for the identified group through the use of specialized data queries, dialing, or contact campaigns. For telephonic disease management programs, this may mean designing dialing campaigns used by predictive dialing software that will automatically dial the person's number, presents the identified patient, dials the patient, then displays the member chart to the disease manager. This technology is well-understood in sales organizations, but is not generally used by commercial disease management companies. Only the largest scale companies will employ this technology.

Population managers will make use of query tools that use clinical information system data elements to produce a list of patients to contact over a given time period. The results of the targeting are mapped against connectivity expectations and also compared to the expected clinical and financial objectives of the program.

DISEASE MANAGEMENT ACCREDITATION DOCUMENTATION SPECIALIST

The emergence of disease management has spawned no less that three accreditations. The National Commission of Quality Assurance (NCQA), the Joint Commission on Accreditation of Healthcare Organizations (JCAHO), and the Utilization Review and Accreditation Commission (URAC) all provide disease management accreditations, and although there are similarities in expected program design and content, there are also significant differences. This has spawned the need for persons who are experienced disease managers to become documentation specialists. This role includes ensuring that the disease management program has the proper documentation, processes, content, and overall design to meet accreditation criteria.

The output of the documentation specialist is many pages in many binders that are organized per the accrediting agency's requirements. The binders will contain standard operating procedures; program content such as patient identification algorithms, assessments, interventions, written patient and physician communications, and program goals; and examples of quality improvement initiatives. This requires above-average knowledge of disease management program design and excellent communication and organizational skills. Quite often, this role also requires extensive interaction with the agency reviewers, which requires skills in diplomacy, presentation, and relationship building.

Because the certification length of time varies, the role may last 8 to 10 months and then not be needed again for 1 to 3 years. If the disease management program desires to maintain all certifications, then the role is necessarily a full-time position because of the continual need to gather information, then undergo the site visit and certification process.

CUSTOMER SERVICE

Almost all of the larger scale disease management programs have a customer service component. Customer service representatives provide nonclinical administrative support to the disease managers. These duties include receiving and routing inbound calls from patients and physicians, mailing or faxing materials, conducting nonclinical assessments with patients, and performing routine data entry into the clinical information system. The customer service representative is more likely to be used in call center environments. Educational preparation requires at least a high school diploma and, in some cases, training in medical terminology or clinical practice management.

Customer service representatives must have excellent communication and customer skills. They are often the first voice that represents the disease management program, therefore playing a vital role in forming a positive first impression.

CHALLENGE QUESTIONS

1. Should a licensed practical nurse be allowed to perform medical screening? Conduct assessments? Provide health education?

2. What is the logical place in disease management for other professions, such as social work, exercise physiology, financial counseling, or the clergy?

CHAPTER 15

Understanding the Role of Basic Health Behaviors

As I see it every day you do one of two things: Build health or produce disease in yourself.

Adelle Davis

OVERVIEW

The purpose of this chapter is to propose a model for disease management practice that acknowledges a threefold approach to patients that includes medical appropriateness and separates the contribution of basic health behaviors to condition-specific behaviors. The model makes an assumption that the basic health behaviors listed at the beginning of this chapter play a significant role in overall health. The model also recognizes that medical care plan appropriateness is a critical piece of the overall picture. Lastly, condition-specific behaviors, such as examining feet for signs of infection or weighing daily for signs of fluid overload, are also important, but may be less effective when the patient lacks basic health-behavior habits.

Basic Health Behaviors

1. Understand and follow your doctor's plan of care.
2. Take medications as prescribed.
3. Follow recommended health screening.
4. Get adequate sleep.
5. Keep a healthy weight and eat right.
6. Get adequate exercise.
7. Drink alcohol in moderation.

131

8. Manage stress.

9. Avoid tobacco.

10. Prevent accidents.

[One area of] great importance is the long-overdue acceptance of the reality that the genesis of ill health and disease involves many factors other than germs and genes. In addition to nutritional, environmental, and occupational factors, there are life situations and experiences that all too frequently predispose, precipitate, and perpetuate the manifestation of the patient's underlying disorder. For too long, aided and abetted by such ill-founded ideas as Diagnostic Related Groups (DRGs), the public, its health statisticians and, too often, many physicians have come to believe that diseases are "things"; they are reified artificially. We now seem to have a body-shop, nuts and bolts, pills and procedures model of medicine and health services. We should never forget as the late Sir Austin Bradford Hill, the doyen of medical statistics, warned us: "Health statistics represent people with the tears wiped off." For too long medicine and its statistical systems have relied on the outmoded 17th century reductionism view of the human condition. The new physics and quantum mechanics have changed the rest of scientific thinking. Now medicine must catch up.[1]

DISEASE MANAGEMENT PROGRAM DESIGN

Disease management as it is currently delivered may be overengineered. This point is readily accepted by program designers, but their response is predictable. In defense, they point back to the expectations of program sponsors to cover all the bases, prove value, and represent best practices. Adding to the high expectations, disease management programs have been designed by people who are capable of designing complex programs—highly capable health care providers, scientists, analytical thinkers, and excellent diagnosticians. All these factors and probably a few more have resulted in 30 to 50 question assessments, hundreds of interventions, frequent calls or contacts, and reams of workbooks. One is left wondering if there may be a simpler, more elegant solution that will help improve health status.

First, a short explanation of where the science of disease management design is today will help to explain the reasoning behind this situation. Traditional disease management programs provide interventions that are primarily condition based and are steeped in the associated best practices. Diabetes disease management programs are extensions of the practice guidelines that call for standards of care such as obtaining a dilated retinal examination or obtaining a Hba1c at certain intervals. The guidelines make mention of the lifestyle-habit impact on diabetes and suggest potential strategies to improve them if needed. The unfortunate truth is that lifestyle aspects are not always assigned the proper status in the program design.

**Figure 15.1   Relationship Between Basic Elements of the
Disease Management Approach**

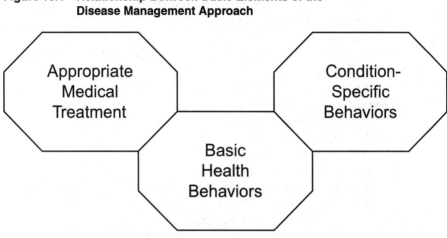

Figure 15.1 provides a graphic explanation of the relationship between these elements. The intent of the diagram is to reinforce that basic health behaviors form the basis of the overall approach. Without those intact, the best medical treatment or condition-specific behaviors are far less effective.

Two brief scenarios will help to illustrate this point further.

Scenario 1

73-year-old man with COPD, hypertension, osteoarthritis, and heart failure.

His basic health habits include:

1. Keep a healthy weight and eat right.
    a. Eats whatever he wants.
    b. Likes to have peanuts while watching football. Tries not to use the salt shaker, but has to use it when he has his steak two to three times per week.
    c. Is about 30 pounds over his recommended weight.
    d. Does not intend to lose weight by dieting.
2. Is as active as possible.
    a. Enjoys snowmobiling with his friends, but is otherwise sedentary.
    b. Hip and knee pain prevent walking without pain for more than 100 feet.

3. Manages stress.
   a. Has significant family strife around him.
   b. Daughter recently passed away.
   c. Is a widower.
   d. Coping mechanism is to lash out when family subjects are raised.
   e. Will occasionally cry when thinking about his wife.
4. Gets regular medical screening.
   a. Doesn't know what screening is necessary and will not seek it.
5. Avoids tobacco.
   a. No longer smokes cigarettes.
   b. Has an 80 pack per year history.
   c. Ten cartons of unfiltered Camel cigarettes are stored in his pantry.
6. Consumes moderate amounts of alcohol.
   a. Has two to four mixed drinks per day. Starts at 4 P.M. sharp.
   b. Sometimes has many more when emotions are running high.
7. Prevents accidents.
   a. Doesn't wear his seat belt.
   b. Takes care in all other areas.
8. Follows the doctor's plan of care.
   a. Favorite saying: "Doctors are only licensed to practice."
   b. Will consider what the doctor says, but will follow his own rules when he either doesn't understand the instructions or doesn't feel like following the instructions.
9. Takes all medications as directed.
   a. Takes all medications as long as he has them.
   b. Will allow medications to run out for weeks at a time, especially his blood pressure medications. He suspects they don't work.
10. Gets adequate sleep.
    a. Sleeps 7 hours a night, but wakes four to five times to use bathroom.

His condition-specific behaviors are:

1. COPD
   a. Uses oxygen by nasal cannula.
   b. Has appropriate inhaler.
2. Hypertension
   a. Prescribed appropriate medications for age and clinical status.

3. Osteoarthritis
   a. Occasionally takes his prescribed medication for joint pain.
4. Heart failure
   a. Rarely weighs himself.
   b. Doesn't keep a log.
   c. Is on the correct medication regime.

In this first scenario, the data and opportunity are rich to intervene in the basic behaviors. Focusing on the condition-specific behaviors may be futile. His treatment plan appears to be reasonable. In this case, the disease manager appropriately emphasizes improving basic health behavior patterns instead of teaching about COPD or heart failure. The patient's issues are far more fundamental than that. The shaded area of Figure 15.2 indicates the area on which the disease manager would focus.

Scenario 2
68-year-old woman with diabetes, hypertension, and osteoporosis.

Her health habits include:

1. Keep a healthy weight and eat right.
   a. Eats a balanced diet for the most part.
   b. Tends toward vegetarian for weeks at a time.
   c. Rarely eats sweets.

Figure 15.2   Basic Health Behaviors Emphasized

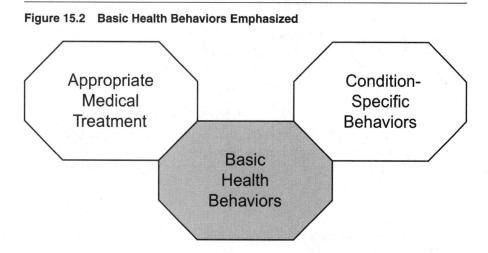

  d. Is 5 pounds under recommended weight.

  e. Has maintained this weight plus or minus 5 pounds for the last 15 years.

2. Is as active as possible.

  a. Is a mall walker 5 days a week.

  b. Is a member of a weekly bowling league.

3. Manages stress.

  a. No significant life stresses.

  b. Lives with husband of 45 years.

  c. Financial situation is stable.

4. Gets regular medical screening.

  a. Follows recommended screening for her age and gender.

  b. Reads *Prevention* magazine.

5. Avoids tobacco.

  a. Does not smoke.

6. Consumes moderate amounts of alcohol.

  a. Has an occasional glass of wine.

7. Is safe.

  a. Wears her seat belt.

  b. Is mindful of household accident potential.

8. Follows the doctor's plan of care.

  a. Writes down her physician's instructions.

  b. Keeps a list of her current medications handy at all times.

  c. Follows her doctor's instructions to the best of her ability.

9. Takes all medications as directed.

  a. Has a pill reminder box.

  b. Rarely forgets to take her medication.

10. Gets adequate sleep.

  a. Sleeps 8 hours a night.

  b. Uses bathroom 1 time per night.

Her condition-specific behaviors are:

1. Diabetes

  a. Tries to check her blood glucose on a weekly basis, but will sometimes skip several weeks.

  b. Has older blood glucose monitor that is heavily technique dependent.

  c. Checks her feet for red spots, but not sure why this is important.

  d. Not taking an ACE inhibitor.

2. Hypertension
   a. Does not monitor her blood pressure at home; only checks during physician visits.
3. Osteoporosis
   a. Not on a bone-building agent despite a recent abnormal bone density test.

This woman has the reverse issues of the man in the first scenario. Her attention to basic health behaviors is laudable, but there are a few treatment issues and behaviors that could be addressed. This scenario also points out the fine line between the appropriateness of medical management and health behaviors. Figure 15.3 represents that the woman is doing her best to do the right things, but there are some elements of medical treatment that need to be addressed. Disease managers should be mindful of this balance and create their plans and set goals in areas that will have the most impact on the person's health.

The remaining chapters in this section provide information relating to each of these behaviors and suggest strategies to help patients to move toward a better approach to their basic health behaviors. The chronic illness section provides information about key medical treatment and condition-specific behaviors.

Figure 15.3   Disease Management Approach Emphasizing Appropriate Medical Treatment and Condition-Specific Behaviors

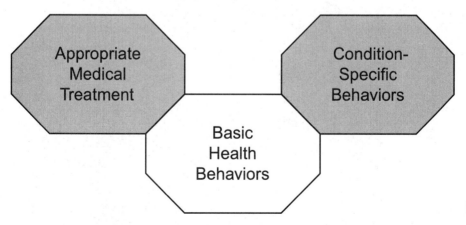

CHALLENGE QUESTIONS

1. There are 10 basic health habits mentioned in this chapter. Are there more?

2. Are basic health habits more important than the other aspects of care?

3. What should a disease manager do when a patient doesn't want to improve their basic health habits?

Endnotes

1. White, Kerr L. *Reflections on the Past and Challenges for the Future.* Hyattsville, MD: The U.S. National Committee on Vital and Health Statistics, 2000.

CHAPTER 16

Understand and Follow
the Plan of Care

One has a greater sense of intellectual degradation after an
interview with a doctor than from any human experience.

Alice James

———— OBJECTIVES ————

1. Describe common problems with understanding and following the plan of care.
2. Describe three methods used to optimize the understanding and adherence to the plan of care.

OVERVIEW

The disease manager is constantly in the position to explain what just happened at the doctor's office. Even though they weren't there physically, there is usually enough information to start the necessary translation for the patient. Commonly, the misunderstandings revolve around reasons for tests, uses for medications, and what the treatment expectations should be for the given treatments. This chapter outlines the case for the challenge of understanding and following the plan of care, and offers strategies for disease managers to make the patient–physician communication more efficient.

RELATIONSHIP BETWEEN UNDERSTANDING
AND CLINICAL OUTCOMES

The likelihood of understanding the plan of care after a visit with the doctor is quite low. The odds are against the patient who is not prepared to participate in their health care in a way that results in clearly articulated instructions that will be remembered, understood, and embraced. Strong evidence exists that optimal adherence to the plan of care is positively correlated with physician–patient relationships,[1] which leads to better health outcomes. Specifically, the outcomes affected were, in descending order of frequency, emotional health, symptom resolution, function, physiologic measures (i.e., blood pressure and blood sugar level), and pain control.[2]

One can draw the same conclusion with the disease manager–patient relationship. Disease managers focus on promoting self-management skills and are thus dependent on using instructional and motivational skills to ensure adherence to the recommendations. In one study examining the effect of communication styles with self-management adherence, there was strong positive association with communication style rather than substance of the visit.[2] It seems as if the burden on following instructions rests squarely on both the sender and the receiver of health care. The purpose of this chapter is to identify the issues that contribute to the lack of plan-of-care understanding and provide strategies for disease managers to use with their patients.

THE ISSUES

It may be helpful to understand what the data is showing about the reality of health-related instructions.

With respect to information:[3]

1. In 65 percent of encounters, internists underestimated their particular patient's desire for information; in only 6 percent did they overestimate.
2. Patients can be divided into seekers (80 percent) and avoiders (20 percent) concerning information, with seekers coping better with more information and avoiders with less.
3. Of 1,012 women with breast cancer attending hospital oncology clinics:[4]
   • 22 percent wanted to select their own cancer treatment.
   • 44 percent wanted to select their treatment collaboratively with their doctors.
   • 34 percent wanted to delegate this decision making to their doctors.
   • 42 percent of women believed they had achieved their preferred level of control in decision making.
4. The time spent in giving instructions is 1 minute out of a 20-minute visit, not 9 minutes as doctors thought.[4]
5. A difference occurs between what type of information the patients want versus what doctors give.[5] The two disagree over the relative importance of imparting different types of medical information. Patients place the highest value on information about prognosis, diagnosis, and causation of their condition while doctors overestimate their patient's desire for information concerning treatment and drug therapy.
6. Fifty to 60 percent of information given to patients is recalled by the patient. For those who remember more, they may suppress or dismiss the

instructions because of a disagreement with the doctor's approach or a trust factor.[6]

7. The actual plan of care experiences a 50 percent adherence. Fifty percent do not adhere to a plan of care.[6]

With respect to the amount of information given by physicians:[5]

1. Physicians give little information to their patients.
2. Most patients want their doctors to provide more information than they do.
3. Physicians overestimate the extent to which they accomplished the following key tasks in explanation and planning: discussing the risks of medication, discussing the patient's ability to follow the treatment plan, and eliciting the patient's opinion about medication prescribed.
4. Despite a lack of basic knowledge prior to the consultation and a strongly expressed desire to gain information concerning their illness, the majority of patients did not obtain even basic information concerning the diagnosis, prognosis, causation, or treatment of their condition.
5. Doctors' instructions to patients when prescribing drugs found no discussion at all in 20 percent of cases, no information about the name or purpose of the drug in 30 percent, no mention of the frequency of doses in 80 percent, or the length of the course in 90 percent.
6. Between 10 to 90 percent of patients prescribed drugs by their doctors (with an average of 50 percent) do not take their medicine at all or take it incorrectly.
7. Physician recommendations are not followed 20 to 30 percent of the time in nonacute illness, 30 to 40 percent of the time in medications for illness prevention, 50 percent of the time for long-term medications, and 72 percent of the time for diet.

With respect to the language and vocabulary used to instruct:[6]

1. The use of technical language (e.g. "febrile, edema, palliative") and medical shorthand (e.g. "history, negative, positive, normal range") was a barrier to communication in more than half of the 800 visits studied. Mothers were confused by the terms used by doctors, yet rarely asked for clarification of unfamiliar terms.
2. Doctors and patients engage in a "communication conspiracy." In only 15 percent of visits where unfamiliar terms were used did the patient admit that they did not understand.[7] Doctors, in turn, seem to speak as if their patients understand all that they say. Physicians deliberately use highly technical language to control communication and to limit patient questions. Such behavior occurred twice as often when doctors were under pressure of time.

3. Physicians are well aware of the difficulties patients have in understanding "doctor-ese" in general. Despite this, in their interviews with patients, physicians continue to use terms that they had previously identified were the very ones that they would not expect their patients to understand.

WORKING FOR BETTER DOCTOR–PATIENT COMMUNICATION

Apparently, patients cannot always depend on their physician to deliver an articulate, meaningful message that will be clearly understood. For this reason, the patient must assume that they will need to take on the role of investigative reporter when receiving instructions from their clinician. There are several proven methods that have shown promise.

Visit Agenda

The first method is the visit agenda. In this method, the patient writes up what they expect from the visit, including issues that are most important and what their treatment goals should be. See Figure 16.1 for an example of a visit agenda. The patient should hand one copy of this agenda to the front office to

---

Figure 16.1   Clinic Visit Agenda

For: Wilma Murphy

Appointment date and time: December 3, 2004, 10:00 A.M.

Primary reason(s) for making appointment:

Refill diabetes medications.

Have right foot checked for sore spot.

Questions for the doctor:

How can I stop taking insulin?

It seems like the rest of my friends are taking different ones for the same problem. Am I on the right medications?

Why isn't the red spot going away on my foot?

My health goals are:

Be on as few medications as possible.

Keep my feet healthy.

Lose a little weight.

Figure 16.2   Patient-Centered Instruction Sheet

For: Wilma Murphy

Appointment date and time: December 3, 2004, 10:00 A.M.

Physician conclusions are that:

Insulin is required until the weight comes down to at least 150 lbs, blood glucose reading is consistently below 126 mg/dl before breakfast, and the Hba1c readings are below 7 percent.

The red spots are early signs of pressure sores and could become blisters without proper foot care. This could lead to infection and more serious consequences if not addressed.

The medications are just right for the range of medical problems.

The physician recommends:

Get the following lab tests done—Hba1c, lipid panel, liver panel, mammogram

Medications—no changes

Instructions—read and follow handouts regarding weight loss, foot care, and blood glucose control

See me when:

There is a worsening in any of your symptoms

In 3 months

insert it into the medical chart. Doing this allows the intake nurse to clarify items on the agenda and possibly answer some questions on behalf of the physician. The physician is then able to review the agenda prior to the visit, review medical chart details, and begin the visit with a common understanding.

Patient-Centered Instruction

The second method is the patient-centered instruction sheet. This idea is synonymous with action plans or patient instruction sheets, but has a more open-ended and flexible format. See Figure 16.2 for an example. The purpose of the patient-centered instruction sheet is for the patient to leave the room with a clear understanding of what the physician just said. With this in hand, the patient can refer to it weeks later to refresh their memory. Having these instructions does not absolutely guarantee adherence to the instructions, however. Sticking to the plan requires self-discipline, motivation, support, and agreement with the viewpoint of the instructions.

Tracking

The last method is in the purview of the disease manager and has to do with adherence and persistence. It is called tracking, monitoring, or reminder messaging. Other chapters in this book have covered aspects of adherence, such as behavior-change techniques, taking medications, and following health screening recommendations. Given the best of all worlds—where a patient has developed a trusting relationship with their physician, uses a visit agenda, and has written instructions—the follow through is all important. The disease manager's role is to build on patient and physician communication to ensure that there is optimal self-management between office visits. Not everyone needs to be tracked all the time, but most patients need it at some time or another. It is for this reason that flexible monitoring methods should be put into place.

Here are a few tenets to keep in mind when performing tracking activities:

- The degree of physician–patient understanding will influence the intensity of contacts.
- The purposes of tracking are to check in, clarify issues, and establish progress.
- Patients will lie about how they are doing when they are not living up to preestablished agreements. The guilt of not doing is too great. They realize the contradictory behavior. Allow for this by admitting to the patients that there are no perfect patients.
- Emphasize beneficial over risky behaviors. Doing this may compel the patient to do more that they are not already doing. "I really admire the way you are able to remember to weigh yourself every day."
- Information gleaned from a patient with limited cognition is still valuable and should be considered. Demented persons can communicate pain levels, for instance. Incorporate family members for finer points or observations.
- Be sensitive to the intensity of tracking activity. A good rule of thumb is to decrease tracking activity when there are several no-problem calls in a row. Ask permission to call less frequently.
- Tracking activity influences behavior, but does not change it in itself. There are far more inputs affecting a patient's life than a physician or a disease manager. Acknowledging that in conversations helps both parties open up the discussion to other influences in their lives.

CHALLENGE QUESTIONS

1. What is the best mechanism for a disease manager to improve the communication between patient and physician?
2. To what degree does physician style play in health outcomes?
3. Is there any problem with disease managers falling into the same communication trap as the physicians?

Endnotes

1. Stewart, M. A. "Effective Physician-Patient Communication and Health Outcomes: A Review." *Canadian Medical Association Journal* 152, no. 9 (May 1, 1955):1423–1433.

2. Heisler, M. "The Relative Importance of Physician Communication, Participatory Decision Making, and Patient Understanding in Diabetes Self-Management." *Journal of General Internal Medicine* 17, no. 4 (April 1, 2002):243–252.

3. Waitzkin, H. "Doctor-Patient Communication: Clinical Implications of Social Scientific Research." *Journal of the American Medical Association* 252, no. 17 (November 2, 1984): 2441–2446.

4. Degner, L. F., Kristjanson, L. B., Bowman, D., Sloan, B. A., Carriere, K. C., O'Neil, J., Bilodeau, B., Watson, P., Mueller, B. "Information needs an decision on preferences in women with breast cancer." *Journal of American Medical Association* 277, no. 18 (May 14, 1997):1485–92.

5. Korsch, B. M. "Gaps in Doctor–Patient Communication. 1: Doctor–Patient Interaction and Patient Satisfaction." *Pediarics* 42, no. 5 (November 1, 1968):855–871.

6. McKinlay, J. B. "Who Is Really Important—Physician or Patient?" *Journal of Health Social Behavior* 16, no. 1 (March 1, 1975):3–11.

7. Tuckett, D. A. "A New Approach to the Measurement of Patients' Understanding of What They Are Told in Medical Consultations." *Journal of Health Social Behavior* 26, no. 1 (March 1, 1985):27–38.

CHAPTER 17

Take Medications as Prescribed

————— OBJECTIVES —————

1. List at least three reasons for medication nonadherence in HIV/AIDS patients and explain why this is an important phenomena to observe.
2. List at least three general themes contributing to medication nonadherence.
3. Describe several special considerations given to elderly patients.

OVERVIEW

Taking medications as prescribed is a challenge for many patients with chronic illness. There are many opportunities for a disease manager to make a significant difference in the clinical outcomes in the area of medication adherence. The purpose of this chapter is to provide the disease manager mechanisms for identifying, then approaching, patients who have issues remembering to take their medications.

Much medication adherence research work has been done in the recent past. Researchers are especially interested in studying populations whose treatment requires strict medication adherence. These populations include, but are limited to, persons with depression, schizophrenia, HIV/AIDS, hypertension, heart failure, asthma, and diabetes. The conclusions from these studies have shed light on this rather complex behavior. Other interesting areas of research are medication adherence and the elderly and the role of the pharmacist in promoting adherence.

MEDICATION ADHERENCE AND HIV/AIDS

HIV/AIDS medication adherence research is particularly useful to the disease manager because it provides insight into the most basic issues. Persons

147

with HIV/AIDS require a strict regime of antiretroviral medications to stave off the virus by keeping their immune systems healthy.

In the mid 1990s, a promising treatment regime was developed for persons with HIV/AIDS called highly active antiretroviral therapy (HAART). Normally this regime calls for two to four medications that are taken throughout the day—sometimes up to four times per day. Years later, it is clear that HAART treatment works well. Patients who stay with the treatment are living an almost-normal life expectancy. The problem with HAART is that it is hard to stay with the program because of side effects, concerns about confidentiality, and emotional issues; therefore, medication doses are missed.

GENERAL MEDICATION ADHERENCE THEMES

Medication adherence studies across multiple conditions point to common themes that sound much like what can happen to anybody during a usual day. Patients say that they simply forgot, were away from their home, missed a dose because they were sleeping, were too ill, were too busy, had a change to their medication routine, or were having side effects.

Physician characteristics also play an important role in medication adherence. One study found that the number of patients seen per week and scheduling a follow-up appointment after prescribing a new medication had a positive affect on medication adherence.[1] Another common medication adherence factor is the complexity of the medication regime. Physicians should do everything in their power to simplify where possible the drug regimens of their patients. This is particularly important in the elderly who are more easily confused. This is also true for the younger population. Research is pointing to improved adherence when the complexity is decreased.[2] Disease managers can provide this kind of feedback to their patients and physicians if medication adherence issues become a pattern with certain physicians.

MEDICATION ADHERENCE AND THE ELDERLY

The elderly have their own issues with medication adherence. Because they often have the dual problem of multiple medications and diminishing memory, remembering to take their medications can be a constant challenge. For instance, older persons will often rely on the pattern of their day to remember to take their medications rather than time. They may tell the disease manager that they take their pills before breakfast, when they pick up the mail, and after the evening news is over.

Moreover, this situation goes past not remembering to take their medications. Other common issues include refusing to take medications, discontinuing their medications, or reducing the dose of the medication.[3] Disease managers must be on the lookout for factors leading to this behavior such as distrust in the prescriber or the medication itself, fear of the medication, cost, adverse reactions, or not being convinced that the medication will benefit them. Other reasons for lack of medication adherence include that the elderly will increase their dosage, take a drug "holiday," or will take the medication because the doctor told them so (white-coat compliance), and discontinuing the medication when the effect wears off.

Vermiere found other interesting age-associated factors for medication nonadherence in the elderly[4]:

1. Have generally more problems with cognition.
2. Have vision or dexterity deficits.
3. Have low reading level, and because English may be their second language, communication may be misinterpreted. The word "once" in Spanish refers to the number eleven, for instance. So an instruction that reads "once a day" could be interpreted as eleven times a day.
4. Generational differences in beliefs on finances, the work ethic, and a confidence in government or medical assistance.

The elderly are also particularly susceptible to adverse reactions to medications due to compromises in gastrointestinal, hepatic, and renal function. Medication doses may need to be smaller or larger to achieve the desired effect. The impact of not arriving at the right dose may drive several of the issues mentioned in this section. Fouts found the following factors are related to the risk for medication nonadherence[5]:

1. 85 years and older.
2. More than six active chronic medical diagnoses.
3. Decreased kidney function (estimated creatinine clearance <50 mL per minute [0.83 mL per second]).
4. Low body weight or body-mass index.
5. Nine or more medications.
6. More than 12 doses of medication per day.
7. Previous adverse drug reaction.

PHARMACIST ROLE IN MEDICATION ADHERENCE

Pharmacists are often in the position to encourage medication adherence. There are innovative models of community-based pharmacists who are extending their practice into the medication adherence arena.[6] In this model, a pharmacist can pair with a social worker or nurse to identify, then provide, communication, medication reminder instruction, and medication regime evaluation services. This model works well for medication adherence because of the trust that is established between the pharmacist and the patient.[7]

POLYPHARMACY

Polypharmacy is another common issue for medication adherence. A standard definition for when poly-pharmacy is present does not exist, but it can be defined as too many medications or more medication than is needed. In a study by Grant and associates[8], the issue of poly-pharmacy and medication in diabetics was explored. The intent was to show that medication adherence is decreased with the number of total medications. The results of this study showed that medication adherence did not decrease with the number of medications. Instead, the diabetics had lower adherence rates when they had side effects that they didn't know they were going to have or did not have confidence in the ability of the medication to benefit their situation.

MEDICATION ADHERENCE REMINDER DEVICES

An entire industry is devoted to medication reminders. Manufacturers are lining up to devise ways to ensure that patients take their medications on time. Reminder devices come in the form of watches, pill dispensers, pill box timers, vibrating alarms, alarm clocks, timers and alarms, personal digital assistants, pagers, cell phones, and jewelry.

The following list represents common reminder devices. These are presented for reference purposes, and do not necessarily represent the entire choice in medication reminders. A common cost of each is in parentheses.

1. Plastic pill reminder boxes, comes in all manner of configurations. All are 7-day style; some have one to four doses per day ($5–20).
2. Electronic medication dispenser with a day-and-time reminder with circular trays that dispense medication (over $200).
3. Pill box timer, features up to 37 alarms ($50).
4. Seven day/four dose organizer with 31 alarms ($60).
5. Automatic monitored pill dispenser, subscription to monitoring service that reports on pill-taking behavior. Machine dispenses pills, then sends a signal to a central database that can be viewed by approved viewers ($740).
6. Vibrating watch, six alarms to remind patient to take medications ($99).
7. 12-alarm vibrating pager ($75).
8. Beep 'n Tell, medication vial with recording stylus on cap that records pill-taking behavior. ($50).

9. Multialarm pocket reminder, alerts patient to upcoming dosing ($35).
10. Medication reminder with pull-out tray and alarms ($40).
11. Vibrating alarm/travel clock ($35).
12. Key ring six-alarm ring fob ($40).

THE DISEASE MANAGER'S ROLE IN MEDICATION ADHERENCE

Assessing the degree of medication is obviously extremely important, based on the findings discussed in this chapter. The disease manager should assess the degree of medication adherence with every contact. Here is a suggested method to ensure that the medication plan is intact.

Disease manager:	Mr. Jones, let's talk through your medications. Do you have a method to help you remember to take your medications?
Mr. Jones:	Yes, I do. I have a plastic box that holds all my pills. My wife puts them in there every Sunday night. Works pretty well.

The fact that there is a reminder method is good, but this does not assure that Mr. Jones is remembering to take the medications or that Mrs. Jones is putting the right medications in the boxes at the right time.

Disease manager:	That's good, Mr. Jones. Do you think that method is working well with you?
Mr. Jones:	Yes, I rarely if ever forget because I put the box next to my recliner so I can see it all the time. I haven't checked the pill bottles to see if my wife is putting them in there right but she's good at that sort of thing.
Disease manager:	It would be a good idea to go through it one time in case she is unable to help you out one Sunday night. Besides, it's good to have another pair of eyes going through how you take your medications.

Remember, wrong dosing and perceived low benefit are prime reasons why patients will discontinue their medications.

Disease manager:	Mr. Jones, do you think your medications are working? I see here that you are taking five of them.
Mr. Jones:	I suppose so. Not sure about the blood pressure pill—I can't tell any difference. I also think the heart pill is making me sleepy; I started to have to take a nap after I got that one. Sometimes I don't take it when I have to be out doing something. My wife doesn't know that.

Medications for chronic illness rarely have day-to-day benefits. Blood pressure and cholesterol medications work behind the scenes to improve asymptomatic conditions. Patients who are not rewarded with good reports (low blood pressure or normal cholesterol values) and understand that it is the medication keeping the condition in check will do better.

We are also picking up that Mr. Jones is having trouble with his heart pill (a cardio-selective beta blocker called Tenormin). Mr. Jones is reacting to the side effects like many people do—managing around it. Medications that interfere with life's routines is another reason why medication adherence is a real challenge. The disease manager can explain that there are other alternatives such as lowering the dose or changing to another medication that does not have the same effect.

Disease manager:	Mr. Jones, controlling your blood pressure is very important. I suggest that you consider speaking to your doctor about what is happening to you during the afternoon. There are plenty of other options to try that do not have the same effect. Now, let's go through the medications you take on a daily basis. Do you have your list with you to read to me?
Mr. Jones:	Yes, I do.
Disease manager:	Please read them to me, one drug at a time across the entire line. I'll stop you if I don't understand something. Ready to start?
Mr. Jones:	Yes, here we go. Lisinopril 10mg 1 pill in the morning . . . Tenormin 50mg 1 pill in the morning . . . Flomax .8mg 1 pill in the morning . . . Plavix 75mg 1 pill in the morning . . . Metaglip 2.5/500mg 1 pill two times a day . . . and I've been taking an aspirin every day for the past 2 weeks—my golfing buddies take one a day to ward off a heart attack.

Mr. Jones did a good job giving the medications to the disease manager. The addition of the aspirin will do no harm in the absence of bleeding disorders or other hemorrhagic situations, but trying additional medications is not an unusual behavior.

Disease manager:	Thanks, you did a good job giving me your list. Please let your doctor know about your taking aspirin. I don't think there should be a problem with taking it. I looked it up and see that people can take the two medications (plavix and aspirin) together as long as they don't have active stomach ulcers or another bleeding problem. You may

	want to watch out for signs of increased tendency to bleed such as bleeding gums or easy bruising. I recommend that you not start any medications before talking to your doctor because you may get into trouble if you pick the wrong one to add. Tell your doctor even if you want to start taking vitamins or anything that will be taken every day.
Mr. Jones:	OK. I understand. I'll talk to him about it on my next appointment. It's in 3 weeks, I think.
Disease manager:	Five medications can be expensive. Are you able to afford them?
Mr. Jones:	So far so good. It costs me about $300 a month because I don't have good insurance. If it goes much higher, I might be in trouble.

The cost of medications is listed as one of the major reasons to discontinue or temporarily stop medications. The disease manager must keep a constant vigilance over the affordability issue. This can be a sensitive subject, but if it is broached in a caring conversation, it will be appreciated. If cost is an issue, ask the patient to return to their doctor to discuss alternative medications that cost less.

CHALLENGE QUESTIONS

1. How often is it necessary to review medications?
2. What does a disease manager do when the patient can't afford their medications even when they can get generic medications?
3. How can a disease manager create an atmosphere that promotes medication adherence?

Endnotes

1. DiMatteo, M. R. "Physicians' Characteristics Influence Patients' Adherence to Medical Treatment: Results from the Medical Outcomes Study." *Health Psychology* 12, no. 2 (March 1, 1993):93–102.

2. Coutts, J. A., Gibson, N. A., and Paton, J. Y., "Measuring Compliance with Inhaled Medication in Asthma." *Archives of Disease in Childhood* 67 (1992):332–333 and Spector, S. L. "Is Your Asthmatic Patient Really Complying?" *Annals of Allergy, Asthma, and Immunology* 55 (1985):552–556.

3. Larosa, J. H., and Larosa, J. C. "Enhancing Drug Compliance in Lipid-Lowering Treatment." *Archives of Family Medicine* 9, no. 10 (Nov–Dec 2000):1169–75.

4. Vermiere, E., Harashaw, H. M., van Royen, P., Denekens, J. "Patient Adherence to Treatment: Three Decades of Research. A Comprehensive Review." *Journal of Clinical Pharmacy and Therapeutics* 5 (2001):331–342.

5. Fouts, M., Hanlon, J., Pieper, C., Perfetto, E., and Feinberg, J. "Identification of Elderly Nursing Facility Residents at High Risk for Drug-Related Problems." *Consultant Pharmacist* 12 (1997):1103–1111.

6. Diaz, A., Defino, M. "The Importance of a Dedicated Medication Adherence Counselor (MAC); Care Teams Provide Model for Community Care." Conference Abstract, XIII International AIDS Conference, 2001.

7. Slack, M. K., McEwen, M. M., Carter, J. T., and Brueckner, R. L. "Case Management Delivery Model for Pharmacy." *American Journal of Health System Pharmacy* 53, no. 23 (1996): 2860–2867.

8. Grant, R., Devita, N., Singer, D., and Meigs, J. "Polypharmacy and Medication Adherence in Patients with Type 2 Diabetes (Epidemiology/Health Services/Psychosocial Research)." *Diabetes Care* 26, no. 5 (2003):1408–1412.

Follow Recommended Health Screening

OVERVIEW

The U.S. Preventive Services Task Force (USPSTF) is the recognized medical screening body and the one disease management programs use as a basis for their recommendations. There are other recommendations from condition-based agencies such as the American Diabetes Association and the National Heart, Lung, and Blood Institute. The goal of this chapter is to discuss the purpose of health screening, strategies that disease managers can use to encourage screening, and to provide the latest general screening recommendations from relevant organizations.

SCREENING

The purpose of health screening is to provide early detection of a disease or condition that if not addressed will cause morbidity or mortality. The key phrases in this definition are early detection and if not addressed. The mechanics of screening are manifold. Screening can imply many persons at one time, such as blood pressure checks at health fairs, or a case-by-case basis. Whatever the health screen, the initiative must include eligibility requirements, timing requirements, screening technique, screening values, rules for a positive screen, and actions for positive and negative screens.

Some health screens reap great value and some are questionable. Screening for cervical cancer using the PAP test is an extremely effective screening technique for the eligible population. Screening for diabetes using a random blood glucose measurement is not effective given the yield of positive results. Screening recommendations follow a predictable course on their way to becoming a valid recommendation. First, there must be compelling evidence that there is research that meets quality-of-evidence parameters. The USPSTF uses a rigorous methodology to ensure that the evidence for their recommendations is of the highest quality. Second, the evidence must point to a clear benefit to conduct the screening. The degree of benefit is hard to quantify in all circumstances. The benefit of screening for prostate cancer is a function of the value of the information once known and the degree to which something can or should be done about the problem. Third, the screening result should have strategies that are known to reduce or eliminate the problem.

Here are screening criteria followed by most agencies:

The disease must have a significant effect on the quality of life.

Acceptable methods of treatment must be available.

There must be an asymptomatic period during which detection and treatment reduces morbidity and mortality.

Treatment in the asymptomatic phase must yield a therapeutic result.

Tests must be available at a reasonable cost and must be acceptable to the patient.

The incidence of the condition must be sufficient to justify the cost of screening.

The disease manager will be in a position to discuss screening tests. The following list is by no means comprehensive, but represents the common screening recommendations and is adapted from the USPSTF recommendations. Please refer to the USPSTF *Guide to Clinical Preventive Services*, 3rd edition, for a full list.[2]

Aspirin Use for Prevention of Cardiovascular Events

The USPSTF strongly recommends that clinicians discuss aspirin chemoprevention with adults who are at increased risk for coronary heart disease (CHD). Discussions with patients should address both the potential benefits and harms of aspirin therapy.

Breast Cancer

Screening mammography, with or without clinical breast examination, every 1 to 2 years for women aged 40 and older.

Evidence is insufficient to recommend for or against routine clinical breast exam alone to screen for breast cancer.

Evidence is insufficient to recommend for or against teaching or performing routine breast self-examination.

Colorectal Cancer

Strong recommendation that clinicians screen men and women 50 years of age or older for colorectal cancer.

Good evidence exists that periodic fecal occult blood testing (FOBT) reduces mortality from colorectal cancer and fair evidence exists that sigmoidoscopy alone or in combination with FOBT reduces mortality.

Cervical Cancer

Strong recommendation to screen for cervical cancer in women who have been sexually active and have a cervix.

Recommendation against routinely screening women older than age 65 for cervical cancer if they have had adequate recent screening with normal Pap smears and are not otherwise at high risk for cervical cancer.

Recommends against routine Pap smear screening for benign disease in women who have had a total hysterectomy.

Evidence is insufficient to recommend for or against the routine use of human papillomavirus testing as a primary screening test for cervical cancer.

Prostate Cancer

Evidence is insufficient to recommend for or against routine screening for prostate cancer using prostate specific antigen (PSA) testing or digital rectal examination (DRE).

Cholesterol

The USPSTF strongly recommends that clinicians routinely screen men aged 35 years and older and women aged 45 years and older for lipid disorders and treat abnormal lipids in people who are at increased risk of coronary heart disease.

The USPSTF recommends that clinicians routinely screen younger adults (men aged 20 to 35 and women aged 20 to 45) for lipid disorders if they have other risk factors for coronary heart disease.

Screening for lipid disorders include measurement of total cholesterol (TC) and high-density lipoprotein cholesterol (HDL–C).

Coronary Artery Disease

Insufficient evidence exists to recommend for or against screening middle-aged and older men and women for asymptomatic coronary artery disease, using resting elecrocardiography (ECG), ambulatory ECG, or exercise ECG.

Recommendations against routine screening can be made on other grounds for individuals who are not at high risk of developing clinical heart disease.

Routine screening is not recommended as part of the periodic health visit or preparticipation sports examination for children, adolescents, or young adults.

Clinicians should emphasize proven measures for the primary prevention of coronary disease.

Depression

Recommendation for screening adults for depression in clinical practices that have systems in place to assure accurate diagnosis, effective treatment, and follow up.

Evidence is insufficient to recommend for or against routine screening of children or adolescents for depression.

Diabetes

Evidence is insufficient to recommend for or against routinely screening asymptomatic adults for type 2 diabetes, impaired glucose tolerance, or impaired fasting glucose.

Recommendation for screening for type 2 diabetes in adults with hypertension or hyperlipidemia.

Drug Abuse

Insufficient evidence exists to recommend for or against routine screening for drug abuse with standardized questionnaires or biologic assays. Including questions about drug use and drug-related problems when taking a history from all adolescent and adult patients may be recommended on other grounds.

All pregnant women should be advised of the potential adverse effects of drug use on the development of the fetus.

Clinicians should be alert to the signs and symptoms of drug abuse in patients and refer drug-abusing patients to specialized treatment facilities where available.

Family Violence

Insufficient evidence exists to recommend for or against the use of specific screening instruments to detect family violence, but recommendations to include questions about physical abuse when taking a history from adult patients may be made on other grounds.

Clinicians should be alert to the various presentations of child abuse, spouse and partner abuse, and elder abuse.

Hearing Impairment

Screening for older adults for hearing impairment is recommended through periodically questioning them about their hearing, counseling them about the availability of hearing aid devices, and making referrals for abnormalities when appropriate.

Hormone Replacement Therapy

Recommendation against the routine use of estrogen and progestin for the prevention of chronic conditions in postmenopausal women.

Evidence is insufficient to recommend for or against the use of unopposed estrogen for the prevention of chronic conditions in postmenopausal women who have had a hysterectomy.

Human Immunodeficiency Virus

Clinicians should assess risk factors for human immunodeficiency virus (HIV) infection by obtaining a careful sexual history and inquiring about injection drug use in all patients. Periodic screening for infection with HIV is recommended for all persons at increased risk of infection. Screening is recommended for all pregnant women at risk for HIV infection, including all women who live in states, counties, or cities with an increased prevalence of HIV infection.

Hypertension

Strong recommendation that clinicians screen adults aged 18 and older for high blood pressure.

Evidence is insufficient to recommend for or against routine screening for high blood pressure in children and adolescents to reduce the risk of cardiovascular disease.

Glaucoma

Insufficient evidence exists to recommend for or against routine screening for intraocular hypertension or glaucoma by primary care clinicians.

Recommendations to refer high-risk patients for evaluation by an eye specialist may be made on other grounds.

Obesity

Recommendation that clinicians screen all adult patients for obesity and offer intensive counseling and behavioral interventions to promote sustained weight loss for obese adults.

Evidence is insufficient to recommend for or against the use of moderate- or low-intensity counseling together with behavioral interventions to promote sustained weight loss in overweight or obese adults.

Osteoporosis

Recommendation that women aged 65 and older be screened routinely for osteoporosis. The USPSTF recommends that routine screening begin at age 60 for women at increased risk for osteoporotic fractures.

No recommendation for or against routine osteoporosis screening in postmenopausal women who are younger than 60 or in women aged 60 to 64 who are not at increased risk for osteoporotic fractures.

Problem Drinking

Screening to prevent problem drinking is recommended for all adult and adolescent patients. Screening should involve a careful history of alcohol use and/or the use of standardized screening questionnaires.

Routine measurement of biochemical markers is not recommended in asymptomatic persons.

Pregant women should be advised to limit or cease drinking during pregnancy. Although there is insufficient evidence to prove or disprove harms from light drinking in pregnancy, recommendations that women abstain from alcohol during pregnancy may be made on other grounds.

All persons who use alcohol should be counseled about the dangers of operating a motor vehicle or performing other potentially dangerous activities after drinking alcohol.

Rubella

All women of childbearing age should be screened for rubella susceptibility by history of vaccination or by serology.

Thyroid Disease

Routine screening for thyroid disease with thyroid function tests is not recommended for asymptomatic children or adults.

Insufficient evidence exists to recommend for or against routine screening for thyroid disease with thyroid-function tests in high-risk patients, but recommendations may be made on other grounds. Clinicians should remain alert to subtle symptoms and signs of thyroid disease when examining such patients.

Visual Impairment

Vision screening to detect amblyopia and strabismus is recommended once for all children prior to entering school, preferably between ages 3 and 4. Screening for diminished visual acuity with Snellen visual acuity chart is recommended for elderly persons.

Screening for Diabetics[1]

Glycemic control

A1C	<7.0%*
Preprandial plasma glucose	90–130 mg/dl (5.0–7.2 mmol/l)
Peak postprandial plasma glucose	<180 mg/dl (<10.0 mmol/l)
Blood pressure	<130/80 mmHg

Lipids

LDL	<100 mg/dl (<2.6 mmol/l)
Triglycerides	<150 mg/dl (<1.7 mmol/l)[†]
HDL	>40 mg/dl (>1.1 mmol/l)[‡]

*Referenced to a nondiabetic range of 4.0–6.0% using a DCCT-based assay.

[†]Current NCEP/ATP III guidelines suggest that in patients with triglycerides ≥200 mg/dl, the "non-HDL cholesterol" (total cholesterol minus HDL) be utilized. The goal is ≤130 mg/dl (53).

[‡]For women, it has been suggested that the HDL goal be increased by 10 mg/dl.

DISEASE MANAGER'S ROLE IN HEALTH SCREENING

The disease manager identifies screening opportunities, engages in informed and shared decision-making activities, and monitors for adherence to the screening recommendation. Disease management programs may have standard assessments, educational materials, or other methods to identify screening opportunities. If this is so, then screening activities have been built in as a part of the value proposition for the program. Whatever the method of identification, the disease manager will be on the front lines of the screening recommendation.

Once the screening recommendation is identified, there may be a period of questioning the usefulness or candidacy for the screening test. The disease manager will then engage in informed decision-making activities. This process is described in Chapter 10.

If the screening is an integral part of the disease management program, then a mechanism to track completion of the screening test is present. Most of the time, this mechanism manifests itself as a goal to complete. Goal tracking is then the final arbiter of completion of the screening test.

Health screening can be costly if conducted on an individual basis. Cost-effective strategies include media-based awareness program, reminder cards, and Web-based tools that propose screening due for the patient. The disease manager may be asked to author screening materials or at least refer to them in the course of their interactions with the patient.

CHALLENGE QUESTIONS

1. What is the value of screening activities in disease management? Is it really worth it?
2. What is the value of screening to a managed care organization?
3. What are some of the best ways to communicate health screening information to patients?

Resources

Report of the U.S. Preventive Services Task Force, www.ahcpr.gov/clinic/gcpspu.htm. (The U.S. Department of Health and Human Services does not endorse any particular organization or its activities, products, or services.)

American Diabetes Association, http://diabetes.org/homepage.jsp.

Endnotes

1. American Diabetes Association, "Standards of Medical Care for Patients with Diabetes Mellitus: American Diabetes Association Clinical Practice Guidelines." *Diabetes Care* 26 (2003): S33–S50.
2. U.S. Preventative Services Task Force, *Guide to Clinical Preventive Services*, 3rd Edition, periodic updates, Publication No. App1P02-0001 (2002).

CHAPTER 19

Get Adequate Sleep

─────── **OBJECTIVES** ───────

1. Describe the burden of sleep disorders for persons with chronic illness.
2. List two common sleep disorders and detail strategies disease managers can use to help their patients.

OVERVIEW

The notion of sleep health is not a common one, yet it is important for any disease manager. This chapter highlights what patients with chronic disease already know; poor sleep affects all aspects of health, and improving sleep health potency impacts overall health.

SLEEP: PART OF THE CARE PLAN

Sleep is an essential aspect of health. There is no substitute for a good night's sleep. When a person is sleep deprived, there is a fundamental shift in judgment, mental acuity, energy level, and metabolic functions. For these reasons, the disease manager must pay careful attention to sleep health as a part of the overall care plan.

Normal sleep ranges are between 6 to 8 hours; some people need fewer, some more. The best measure of adequate sleep is the subjective measure of wakefulness. Ideally, a person wakes refreshed, has full energy through the day, and then begins to feel tired 1 to 2 hours before retiring.

Everyone has trouble sleeping at some point during their life due to life stresses, changes in schedules, illness, injury, or sleep disorders. The nonsleep disorder conditions, as well as the sleep disorders, are treatable to some extent.

The impact of sleep disorders is staggering. Consider the following consequences of sleepiness:

- Between 1989–1993 there were approximately 56,000 people a year killed because they fell asleep at the wheel.[1]
- Younger persons have documented lapses in concentration, memory, and scholastic achievement due to sleep deprivation.[2]
- In the workplace, sleepiness contributes to lost productivity, accidents, and death.[3]

Disordered sleep negatively impacts those with chronic disease, namely hypertension, vascular disease, heart attacks, and stroke. There is a growing body of evidence that sleep apnea may either cause or worsen hypertension and insulin sensitivity. Because a large proportion of persons with sleep apnea are obese, the potential impact is high.

GENERAL SLEEP HEALTH

Healthy sleep is vital to all aspects of a person's well-being. All persons have a unique sleep/wake cycle (circadian rhythm) that when not disturbed, maintains a healthy rhythm both physically and emotionally. The circadian rhythm is a hormonally driven biologic clock that causes a person to want to sleep for about a third of a day; about 8 hours.

Here is a list of health actions sleep experts recommend for optimal sleep:

- Have a regular bedtime (the same time every day).
- Avoid naps or make them no longer than 20 minutes.
- Do not have caffeine after lunch.
- Do not have alcohol at night. Consume only a small amount; it is a recipe for disturbed sleep.
- Have a regular bedtime routine.
- Do not stay in bed trying to go to sleep when you are not tired. Get up and do something quiet like reading and try again when you feel tiredness coming on.
- Take care to avoid medications that may disturb sleep. Certain cold preparations cause agitation, for instance.
- Be active during the day. A physically active person usually does not have sleep problems.
- Persons with chronic pain should consult their physicians about pain control, physical therapy, or recommended sleep positions.

The primary sleep disorders are sleep apnea, narcolepsy, and insomnia.

Sleep Apnea

Sleep apnea is characterized as sudden interruptions in sleep. Persons with sleep apnea wake suddenly, gasping and choking for air without knowing why. They may have 20 to 30 episodes per hour in between loud snoring and fitful sleep. These apnic events are almost always accompanied by snoring, but there are those who do not snore and still have sleep apnea. Because sleep is chaotic, the normal sleep cycles are not present, and the person is left with a sleep debt that is not repaid.

Sleep apnea is more common than officially diagnosed. Estimates are that up to 18 million people in the United States have sleep apnea.[4] It is more common in men than women and, for unknown reasons, young African Americans under 18 years old.

There are two types of sleep apnea: central and obstructive. Central sleep apnea is caused by faulty signals from the central nervous system and is far less common than obstructive sleep apnea. Obstructive sleep apnea is caused by blockage due to internal anatomical reasons such as a deviated septum or external reasons such as obesity. In others, the neck and throat muscles relax to such an extent that the airway loses its integrity, thus preventing normal airway exchange.

Because the rates of obesity have increased in recent years, obstructive sleep apnea is becoming more common. When an obese person sleeps, the mass of adipose tissue flattens out across the abdomen, chest, and neck region, causing the airway passage to narrow. Sometimes, it is only the sleep partner who is aware of the apnic events. This is especially true for those who take sleeping aids or ingest alcohol.

Assessment of Sleep Apnea

Through a series of questions, the disease manager can quickly assess whether the person may be suffering from obstructive sleep apnea.

Q: Do you have trouble with sleepiness compared to those around you?

The presence of sleepiness is an effect of obstructive sleep apnea. This question helps to acknowledge the presence of unusual sleepiness and opens the person to further investigation.

Q: Do you fight falling asleep when you are listening, sitting, or driving?

This is a general question and does not indicate a root problem. The purpose of the question is to open the dialogue.

Q: Do you find yourself falling asleep when there are people around you?

Many persons with sleep apnea have a constant problem with sleep debt and succumb to the habit of sleeping when they should be fully awake and energized. The mention of sleeping around people is meant to make the point that the disorder is taking control over their time.

Q: When you are sleeping, do you have a pattern of waking suddenly, perhaps gasping or choking for air?

Gasping and choking for air while sleeping indicates disordered sleep and may indicate sleep apnea. Notice the use of the word "pattern." Waking up once or twice with these symptoms is less problematic than a more frequent pattern.

Q: Does your sleep partner say that when they watch you sleep, you snore loudly, seem to stop breathing for a few seconds, then return to sleep?

The observation of this pattern by another is critical. Try to elicit frequency of these events if possible.

Diagnosis of Sleep Apnea

Diagnosing sleep apnea is challenging because there are many factors that can contribute to disordered sleep. The subjective information collected is an important first step. Sleep centers use Polysomnography, a test that evaluates the sleeping person's body systems. The Multiple Sleep Latency Test measures the time it takes to fall asleep. Persons who fall asleep in less than 5 minutes probably have a sleep debt and thus a disorder. There are other diagnostic tests coming on board and will be made available at sleep clinics.

Narcolepsy

Narcolepsy is a bothersome and potentially serious condition that can manifest in a variety of ways. Most narcoleptics suffer from frequent, daily "sleep attacks"; moments of muscle weakness usually brought on when emotions are running high. Fewer have short sleep episodes, called microsleep, which appears as if the person is awake, but is not; short periods of paralysis that are unexplained, dream-like states while awake; and lastly, limb movements while asleep.

Narcolepsy is relatively rare, and its cause is not well-understood. It is a lifelong disorder, but does not worsen over time. Because the condition severely disrupts a person's sleep, there are many medical, psychological, and social issues. The primary points of concern are accidents and difficulty with social interactions.

Assessment of Narcolepsy

Through a series of questions, narcolepsy may be determined.

Q: Do you experience excessive daytime sleepiness?

All narcoleptics have significant, daily problems with daytime sleepiness. Sometimes these periods end in short naps.

Q: Do you feel like you can't move when you are angry or are laughing, following a heavy meal, or when stressed?

Cataplexy, the inability to move while awake, is a common sign for those with narcolepsy. For most, the cataleptic attack is mild, only lasting a few moments; for others, the attack can last for 30 seconds or more. The head may drop, jaw tightened, and speech may become disorganized, loud, or stuttering.

Diagnosis of Narcolepsy

The signs and symptoms of narcolepsy are sometimes lost over a number of years and attributed to psychological problems. Astute clinicians, those with a sensitivity to narcolepsy, are more inclined to consider this diagnosis earlier in the course. Narcolepsy is often a diagnosis of exclusion. The history of the symptom pattern just mentioned, along with abnormal ECG sleep patterns (abnormal rapid eye movements), and a host of other diagnostic procedures that are designed to rule out related conditions, result in leaving narcolepsy as a logical diagnosis.

Specialists use the Epworth Sleepiness Scale to help diagnose narcolepsy and other related conditions. This scale is readily available on the Internet or in sleep-related texts.

Treatment of Narcolepsy

There are pharmacologic and nonpharmacologic narcolepsy treatments, but no certain treatments. Some persons respond to scheduled sleep treatments that include regular sleep periods and naps throughout the day. An example of a sleep schedule is a nighttime period (11:00 P.M.–7:30 A.M.) and two 15-minute naps before lunch and dinner. Heavy meals and alcohol are not recommended.

Standard medications for narcolepsy include Methylphenidate (Ritalin), Dextroamphetamine (Dexedrine), and Pemoline (Cylert). These act as stimulants, so have the regular cautions for persons who have hypertension, active heart disease, hyperthyroidism, anxiety disorder, and glaucoma.

Insomnia

Insomnia is the most common of all sleep disorders. Insomnia is characterized as pattern daytime sleepiness and extremely light, sometimes fitful sleep, with early morning awakening. Some estimates are that up to a third of all Americans have bouts of insomnia.

Transient insomnia lasts for no longer than 3 days at time, short-term insomnia last for no longer than 3 weeks, and chronic insomnia last for weeks or months. Insomnia symptoms should be present at least 3 days in a week and follow the symptom pattern just mentioned. There is a debate as to whether insomnia is a condition or a result of another underlying condition. Primary insomnia is diagnosed when it is the sole complaint; secondary insomnia, when there is a constellation of symptoms.

There are many aspects of health that are affected by insomnia; it is difficult to provide a comprehensive list. The central theme is that when a person has insomnia, all systems are affected negatively, and until normal sleep patterns are restored, the chances for optimal health are quite limited.

Assessment of Insomnia

Many of the questions in this chapter apply to insomnia. Here are a few more that are useful.

Q: How restful is your sleep?

Insomniacs will say that they "remember" their night sleep and may not have dreams.

Q: Do you wake early, even though you feel you would like more sleep?

Early, tired awakening is a common problem.

Q: How many days per week have you had these symptoms?

This question is used to determine the chronicity of the problem.

Q: Is sleepiness your only problem?

Quite often, the sleepiness is caused by other factors that, when addressed, improve sleep health.

Q: What lifestyle issues could be causing problems with your sleep? (stress, anxiety, pain, medications, alcohol)

Even though all persons have issues that sometimes cause sleep problems, chronic issues should be addressed.

Q: Are you a rotating shift worker?

Shift workers have a high incidence of insomnia because the usual circadian rhythms are not consistent.

Q: Have you caught yourself falling asleep when driving?

This is a safety issue; strong counseling is in order.

Q: Are you withdrawing from caffeine, cigarettes, or medications?

Withdrawing from stimulant-containing substances are common (and temporary) reasons for insomnia.

Diagnosis and Treatment of Insomnia

Sleep experts use the same diagnostic measures mentioned earlier in this chapter. The challenge continues to be early detection, appropriate medical work-up to exclude underlying conditions, and nonpharmacologic and pharmacologic treatment choice.

DISEASE MANAGERS AND SLEEP HEALTH

The best sleep health interventions available to disease managers are not technical and complex. Disease manager interventions include:

- Always be open to the possibility of a sleep disorder.
- Ask about patients' sleep; listen for patterns.
- Consider the fundamental effects of sleepiness on the ability of the person to care for themselves, especially in the attitude department.
- Become knowledgeable about the primary sleep disorders and direct positive screens to sleep specialists.
- Keep lifestyle-related issues in mind when thinking about sleep habits. Exercise, diet, stress, and alcohol all affect sleep patterns.

CHALLENGE QUESTIONS

1. What is the best way for a disease manager to quickly ascertain if a patient is sleep deprived?
2. Aside from falling asleep at the wheel while driving, what are other consequences of sleep deprivation that affect patients with a chronic illness?
3. What are the impacts to the family of the patient with obstructive sleep apnea?

Resources

American Academy of Sleep Medicine, One Westbrook Corporate Center, Suite 920, Westchester, IL 60154; 708-492-0930 or www.aasmnet.org.

National Center for Sleep Disorders Research, National Heart, Lung, Blood Institute, PO Box 30105, Bethesda, MD 20824-0105; 301-251-1222 or www.nhlbi.nih.gov/health/public/sleep/index.htm.

National Sleep Foundation, 1522 K Street, NW, Suite 500, Washington, DC 20005; 202-347-3471 or www.sleepfoundation.org.

The Sleep Well, 702 Marshall Street, Suite 520, Redwood City, CA 94063; 650-365-6492 or www.sleepquest.com.

Society for Light Treatment and Biological Rhythms, PO Box 591687, 174 Cook Street, San Francisco, CA 94159-1687; http://www.sltbr.org. FAX: 415-751-2758.

Endnotes

1. Knipling, R. R., and Wang, J-S. *Crashes and Fatalities Related to Driver Drowsiness/Fatigue.* Research note. Washington, DC: National Highway Traffic Safety Administration, U.S. Department of Transportation, 1994; Findley, L., Unverzagt, M., Guchu, R., Fabrizio, M., Buckner, J., and Suratt, P. "Vigilance and Automobile Accidents in Patients with Sleep Apnea or Narcolepsy." *Chest* 108, no. 3 (1995):619–625; and New York State Task Force on the Impact of Fatigue on Driving. *1994 Telephone Survey on Drowsy Driving: Summary Report.* Albany, NY: Institute for Traffic Safety Management and Research, December 1994.

2. Carskadon, M. A., Rosekind, M. R., Galli, J., Sohn, J., Herman, K. B., and Davis, S. S. "Adolescent Sleepiness During Sleep Restriction in the Natural Environment." *Sleep Res* 18 (1989):115.

3. Dinges, D. F. "An Overview of Sleepiness and Accidents." *Journal of Sleep Res* 4, Supplement 2 (1995):4–14.

4. National Sleep Foundation Web Content: www.sleepfoundation.org/publications/sleepap.cfm.

Keep a Healthy Weight and Eat Right

OVERVIEW

Everyone knows that maintaining a healthy weight and eating right is important. Indeed, there are social expectations to be thin. The negative health impact of weighing too much is on the news at least on a weekly basis. While all of this is true, the number of overweight and obese people is on the rise in alarming proportions. For the disease manager, this issue is especially critical because weight plays a critical role in the effectiveness of their interventions.

The purpose of this chapter is to outline the issues surrounding obesity and to suggest strategies for the disease manager to try with their patients. For the obese person, the outlook for weight loss is not positive. For many, weight control will be a lifelong battle that will have many more losses than victories. It is not for the lack of trying; there are billions spent on weight-loss programs, pills, and other such promises every year.

171

A NATIONAL CRISIS

The number of overweight and obese persons has reached national crisis proportion. Consider the following statistics from the National Center for Health Statistics[1]:

Sixty-four percent of U.S. adults are overweight or obese.

Thirty percent of U.S. adults are obese (body mass index greater than or equal to 30.0).

Percent of adolescents (ages 12–19) who are overweight: 15 percent.

Percent of children (ages 6–11) who are overweight: 15 percent.

Data from the Center for Disease Control[2] reveals the following:

- An obesity epidemic within the U.S. population is portrayed by evidence that in 1991, only 4 of 45 participating states had obesity prevalence rates of 15 to 19 percent and none had prevalence greater than 20 percent.
- By the year 2000, all of the 50 states except Colorado had prevalences of 15 percent or greater with 22 of the 50 states having obesity prevalence as high as 20 percent or greater.
- In 2001, 20 states had obesity prevalences of 15 to 19 percent; 29 states had prevalences of 20 to 24 percent; and one state reported a prevalence more than 25 percent. The prevalence of obesity among U.S. adults increased to 20.9 percent in 2001, a 5.6 percent increase in 1 year and a 74 percent increase since 1991.

The prevalence of overweight and obesity crosses all age, gender, and racial groups. Refer to Table 20.1 for the breakdown.

IMPACT OF OVERWEIGHT AND OBESITY OF HEALTH STATUS

For a long time, there was no convincing scientific evidence that weight affected health status. This is no longer true. As it turns out, the more a person weighs over their normal range, the more likely they are to have a serious chronic condition. The list of conditions affected by weight is long and growing. Here are the primary conditions that, when combined with obesity, are a recipe for high risk and will require intense interventions to reduce weight:

Established coronary heart disease (CHD)

History of myocardial infarction

History of angina pectoris (stable or unstable)

History of coronary artery surgery

Table 20.1   Combined Prevalence of Overweight and Obesity (BMI ≥25.0 kg/m²) Among Adults Age 20 to 80+ Years, By Gender, Race/Ethnicity, and Age: United States, 1960–1994

Gender, race/ethnicity, age 20 years and older, age adjusted	National Health Examination Survey—Cycle I 1960–62 (age 20–74) (%)	National Health and Nutrition Examination Survey I 1971–74 (age 20–74) (%)	National Health and Nutrition Examination Survey II 1976–80 (age 20–74) (%)	National Health and Nutrition Examination Survey 1982–84 (age 20–74) (%)	National Health and Nutrition Examination Survey III 1988–94 (age ≥20) (%)
Both sexes	43.3	46.1	46.0		54.9
Men	48.2	52.9	51.4		59.4
Women	38.7	39.7	40.8		50.7
White men	48.8	53.7	52.3		61.0
White women	36.1	37.6	38.4		49.2
Black men	43.1	48.9	49.0		56.5
Black women	57.0	57.6	61.0		65.8
White, non-Hispanic men			52.0		60.6
White, non-Hispanic women			37.6		47.4

Table 20.1   Combined Prevalence of Overweight and Obesity (BMI ≥25.0 kg/m²) Among Adults Age 20 to 80+ Years, By Gender, Race/Ethnicity, and Age: United States, 1960–1994 (continued)

Gender, race/ethnicity, age 20 years and older, age adjusted	National Health Examination Survey—Cycle I 1960–62 (age 20–74) (%)	National Health and Nutrition Examination Survey I 1971–74 (age 20–74) (%)	National Health and Nutrition Examination Survey II 1976–80 (age 20–74) (%)	National Health and Nutrition Examination Survey 1982–84 (age 20–74) (%)	National Health and Nutrition Examination Survey III 1988–94 (age ≥20) (%)
Black, non-Hispanic men			48.9		56.7
Black, non-Hispanic women			60.6		66.0
Mexican-American men				59.7	63.9
Mexican-American women				60.1	65.9
Age and gender-specific categories					
Men					
20–29	39.9	38.6	37.0		43.1
30–39	49.6	58.1	52.6		58.1
40–49	53.6	63.6	60.3		65.5
50–59	54.1	58.4	60.8		73.0

Table 20.1 Combined Prevalence of Overweight and Obesity (BMI ≥25.0 kg/m²) Among Adults Age 20 to 80+ Years, By Gender, Race/Ethnicity, and Age: United States, 1960–1994 (*continued*)

Age and gender-specific categories			
Men			
60–69	52.9	55.6	57.4	70.3
70–79	36.0	52.7	53.3	63.1
80+	N/A	N/A	N/A	50.6
Women			
20–29	17.0	23.2	25.0	33.1
30–39	32.8	35.0	36.8	47.0
40–49	42.3	44.6	44.4	52.7
50–59	55.0	52.2	52.8	64.4
60–69	63.1	56.2	56.5	64.0
70–74*	57.4	55.9	58.2	57.9
80+	N/A	N/A	N/A	50.1

*Prevalence for age 70 to 74 years only

N/A = Not available

Source: National Heart, Lung, and Blood Institute. *Clinical Guideline on the Identification, Evaluation, and Treatment of Overweight and Obesity in Adults.* Bethesda, MD: NHLBI (1998).

History of coronary artery procedures (angioplasty)

Presence of other atherosclerotic diseases

Peripheral arterial disease

Abdominal aortic aneurysm

Symptomatic carotid artery disease

Type 2 diabetes

Sleep apnea

Any three of the following places a person, overweight or not, into a high absolute risk of heart disease. Overweight or obese persons have an added measure of risk.

Cigarette smoking

Hypertension (systolic blood pressure ≥140 mm Hg or diastolic blood pressure ≥90 mm Hg, or the patient is taking antihypertensive agents)

High-risk LDL-cholesterol (≥160 mg/dL), low HDL-cholesterol (≥35 mg/dL), impaired fasting glucose (fasting plasma glucose of 110 to 125 mg/dL)

Family history of premature CHD (definite myocardial infarction or sudden death at or before 55 years of age in father or other male first-degree relative, or at or before 65 years of age in mother or other female first-degree relative)

Age (men ≥45 years and women ≥55 years or postmenopausal)

Obese patients who have gynecological abnormalities, osteoarthritis, gallstones, and stress incontinence also need interventions, but these combinations are not life threatening.

TREATMENT GOALS

The treatment goals of weight loss and maintenance are to prevent further weight gain, to reduce body weight, and to maintain a lower body weight over the long term.

ASSESSMENT

Overweight and obesity are distinct weight classifications. Body mass index (BMI) is the best method to determine the relative percent of body fat one has. Waist circumference is also closely associated with cardiovascular risk and is used to determine the degree of risk. Tables 20.2 and 20.3 provide detail

Table 20.2   Selected BMI Units Categorized by Inches (cm) and Pounds (kg)

Height in inches (cm)	BMI 25 kg/m^2	BMI 27 kg/m^2	BMI 30 kg/m^2
	Body weight in pounds (kg)		
58 (147.32)	119 (53.98)	129 (58.51)	143 (64.86)
59 (149.86)	124 (56.25)	133 (60.33)	148 (67.13)
60 (152.40)	128 (58.06)	138 (62.60)	153 (69.40)
61 (154.94)	132 (59.87)	143 (64.86)	158 (71.67)
62 (157.48)	136 (61.69)	147 (66.68)	164 (74.39)
63(160.02)	141 (63.96)	152 (68.95)	169 (76.66)
64 (162.56)	145 (65.77)	157 (71.22)	174 (78.93)
65 (165.10)	150 (68.04)	162 (73.48)	180 (81.65)
66 (167.64)	155 (70.31)	167 (75.75)	186 (84.37)
67 (170.18)	159 (72.12)	172 (78.02)	191 (86.64)
68 (172.72)	164 (74.39)	177 (80.29)	197 (89.36)
69 (175.26)	169 (76.66)	182 (82.56)	203 (92.08)
70 (177.80)	174 (78.93)	188 (85.28)	207 (93.90)
71 (180.34)	179 (81.19)	193 (87.54)	215 (97.52)
72 (182.88)	184 (83.46)	199 (90.27)	221 (100.25)
73 (185.42)	189 (85.73)	204 (92.53)	227 (102.97)
74 (187.96)	194 (88.00)	210 (95.26)	233 (105.69)
75 (190.50)	200 (90.72)	216 (97.98)	240 (108.86)
76 (193.04)	205 (92.99)	221(100.25)	246 (111.59)

Table 20.2   Selected BMI Units Categorized by Inches (cm) and Pounds (kg) (*continued*)

Metric conversion formula = weight (kg)/height (m)^2	Nonmetric conversion formula = [weight (pounds)/height (inches)^2] × 704.5
Example of BMI calculation: A person who weighs 78.93 kilograms and is 177 centimeters tall has a BMI of 25: weight (78.93 kg)/height (1.77 m)^2 = 25	Example of BMI calculation: A person who weighs 164 pounds and is 68 inches (or 5′ 8″) tall has a BMI of 25: [weight (164 pounds)/height (68 inches)^2] × 704.5 = 25

Source: National Heart, Lung, and Blood Institute. *Clinical Guideline on the Identification, Evaluation, and Treatment of Overweight and Obesity in Adults.* Bethesda, MD: NHLBI (1998).

Table 20.3   Classification of Overweight and Obesity by BMI, Waist Circumference, and Associated Disease Risks

	BMI (kg/m^2)	Obesity class	Disease risk relative to normal weight and waist circumference	
			Men ≤102 cm (≤40 in) Women ≤88 cm (≤35 in)	>102 cm (>40 in) >88 cm (>35 in)
Underweight	<18.5		—	—
Normal	18.5–24.9		—	—
Overweight	25.0–29.9		Increased	High
Obesity	30.0–34.9	I	High	Very high
	35.0–39.9	II	Very high	Very high
Extreme obesity	≥40	III	Extremely high	Extremely high

Source: National Heart, Lung, and Blood Institute. *Clinical Guideline on the Identification, Evaluation, and Treatment of Overweight and Obesity in Adults.* Bethesda, MD: NHLBI (1998).

on BMI measurement and the classification of overweight versus obesity by BMI and waist circumference.

Given the nature of obesity, the disease manager's assessment must be conducted in an atmosphere of sensitivity and understanding. Often times, patients have been lectured or admonished about their weight and may be on the lookout for another perceived tongue lashing. Here is a weight assessment that is designed to elicit the facts without the feeling of judgment or accusation (once you know that they are overweight or obese through the aforementioned parameters):

Q: What are your concerns about your weight?

Opening up the conversation in this way conveys a sense of support and future teamwork. Because the march toward a healthy weight is long, the patient needs to know they will have a supportive partner.

The concerns may range from cosmetic appearance to functional ability to health-related issues. Be careful to just listen and prompt for more detail if the person requires it. The more concerns the person can volunteer, the more the topic will open up to treatment options.

Q: What are the benefits to being your current weight?

This may seem like a bad question! In fact, this is the best question to ask. The person may answer with some startling opinions like "I am the healthiest at this weight. I once lost 50 pounds and got sick. I felt awful," or they may say, "My friends think I look good."

No matter what the response, listen without flinching. Do not let your own feelings enter into the conversation. Make sure to prompt again for more benefits. Do not let the person say that there are not benefits to being overweight because that is what they are expected to say and does not reflect their true feelings.

Q: What, in your opinion, are your concerns about losing weight?

This question introduces the process of losing weight. This question will probably bring out stories of past failed attempts. Listen for patterns of usual approaches: diet types, food choices, inclusion of other people, length of time on the diet, and results.

Q: What are the benefits to losing weight?

Once you have arrived at this question, the person is far down the thought trail. They have formed in their mind the nature of their situation in a fairly objective manner. This may have happened for the first time in their life. Be a patient listener while they work through the 4 × 4 grid they are now forming in their mind (see Table 20.4 for an example). This grid is called a concerns-and-benefits grid and is meant to elicit information to be used to craft an intervention.

Notice that the answers in the grid in Table 20.4 do not address clinical risk. This person does not raise a concern or benefit relating to their risk of worsening or contracting a chronic condition. There are some persons who would include that answer. The data in these columns are rich in substance and can be used to tailor the education and approach needs of the person for this issue.

Q: What are your motivations, if any, to return to a lower weight?

Using the word "motivation" introduces the person to a sense of promise of a new state of being. If the person says that they are not motivated, then the conversation should return to the concerns-and-benefits discussion until motivation is in evidence. Motivation starts with the belief that there is a better place to be.

In the weight-loss area, motivation is not hard to find. Consider this press report from Atlantic Information Services Managed Care Online News.[3]

As Americans turned to the Web to help kick off a healthy new year, more than 11 million home surfers flocked to health, fitness, and nutrition sites during the week ending Jan. 4, according to recent data from Nielsen//NetRatings, a provider of Internet audience measurement and analysis. The top sites in the health category experienced triple- and double-digit growth, compared with the prior week's levels, the company reports. Weekly traffic to eDiets.com skyrocketed 119% to more than 1 million unique visitors, as compared with 472,000 visi-

Table 20.4   Benefits-and-Concerns Grid

	Concerns	Benefits
Staying the way you are	I can't climb my stairs without being out of breath.	I feel pretty good. My friends don't mind the way I look—I think I look pretty good as well.
Losing weight	I have tried a million diets—none of them have worked. I'm heavier than ever. I can't afford the time or money it will take to lose weight.	I will feel even better. I can fit into clothes that I prefer to wear.

tors during the week ending Dec. 28, reports Nielsen//NetRatings. More than 35% of users, says the firm, accessed a page to receive a free diet profile. Weight Watchers surged 97% to 876,000 visitors from 445,000 visitors during the previous week, according to Nielsen//NetRatings. The company also found that WebMD attracted 853,000 visitors, up 63% from the prior week. The firm notes that 57% of visitors to WebMD went to the Weight Loss Clinic page within the site. Rounding out the top five health, fitness, and nutrition Web sites, Nielsen//NetRatings says, were AOL Health and Yahoo! Health, which grew 59% and 49%, respectively. Traffic to all five sites as a whole increased by 76% week over week from 2.1 million to 3.8 million unique visitors, the firm added.

This provides a snapshot into the numbers of people seeking weight-loss solutions and the zeal in which they do it.

WEIGHT LOSS AND WEIGHT MAINTENANCE

There have been many motivational videos, books, and programs related to weight loss. They have worked to some degree with some people, but the majority are left hanging when life takes over. The skills and techniques required for weight loss are distinct from those to keep the weight off.

Skills needed to initiate weight management are different from those to maintain healthy weight. The disease manager should work through the weight loss process keeping in mind that this is a two-step process—taking and keeping weight off. There is not one best way to lose weight because there is not one person in the world who needs to lose weight! The vast majority of successful weight losers have done it on their own and in their own way.

Here are a few common techniques used by those successful in losing weight:

1. Eat low-glycemic index foods in reasonable portions to maintain a steady state blood glucose. (The glycemic index compares the difference in blood glucose elevation between ingestion of simple carbohydrates and the food in question. Low-glycemic index foods cause the blood glucose to rise slower than high-glycemic index foods.) Doing this curbs hunger as a result of steady insulin levels and causes other metabolic changes to induce weight loss. A list of low-glycemic foods can be found at the end of this section.

2. When possible, eat small frequent meals. Breakfast, mid-morning, lunch, mid-afternoon, dinner, and a bedtime snack is a day full of eating that will lead to weight loss when the proper foods and portions are consumed.

3. Emphasize protein in the diet. Doing this slows the absorption of food.

4. Eat foods that are water filled like fruits and vegetables. A food like a baked pasta dish is denser and likely has a high-glycemic index.

5. Stay as active as possible. Experts recommend 30 minutes per day at least 5 days a week.

6. Stay with it. Persistence is what separates the losers from the gainers. Unsuccessful people use the same techniques as the successful ones, just for much shorter periods of time. Weight loss is a long road, sometimes into the many-months category. Set realistic, long-term goals with many short-term goals in between.

Low-Glycemic Foods

Glycemic index standard = 100%
White bread

High-Glycemic Foods

Glycemic index greater than 100%
- **Grain-based foods**
  Puffed rice
  Cornflakes
  Puffed wheat
  Millet
  Instant rice
  Instant potatoes
  Microwave potato
  French bread
- **Simple sugars**
  Maltose
  Glucose
- **Snacks**
  Tofu ice cream
  Puffed-rice cakes

Glycemic index between 80 and 100%
- **Grain-based foods**
  Grapenuts
  Whole-wheat bread
  Oat bran
  Instant mashed potatoes
  White rice
  Brown rice
  Muesli
  Shredded wheat
- **Vegetables**
  Carrots

Parsnips
Corn
- **Fruits**
  Banana
  Raisins
  Apricots
  Papayas
  Mango
- **Snacks**
  Ice cream (low fat)
  Corn chips
  Rye crisps

Moderate Inducers of Insulin

Glycemic Index Between 50 and 80%
- **Grain-based foods**
  Spaghetti (white or whole wheat)
  Pasta, Other
  Pumpernickel bread
  All-bran cereal
- **Fruits**
  Orange
  Orange juice
- **Vegetables**
  Peas
  Pinto beans
  Kidney beans (canned)
  Baked beans
  Navy beans
- **Simple sugars**
  Lactose
  Sucrose
- **Snacks**
  Candy bar
  Potato chips (with fat)

Reduced Insulin Secretion

Glycemic Index Between 30 and 50%
- **Grain-based foods**
  Barley
  Oatmeal (slow cooking)
  Whole-grain rye bread
  Fruits

Apple
Apple juice
Applesauce
Pears
Grapes
Peaches
- **Vegetables**
Kidney beans (fresh)
Lentils
Black-eyed peas
Chickpeas
Kidney beans (dehydrated)
Lima beans
Tomato soup
- **Dairy products**
Ice cream (high fat)
Milk (skim)
Milk (whole)
Yogurt

WEIGHT LOSS MEDICATIONS

Taking medications for weight loss is not the best weight-loss method; however, there are a select few that may be appropriate for this route. Many medication-based weight-loss treatments exist, but because of the underlying amphetamine-like mechanism of action, it is not unusual to have significant adverse reactions and subsequent removal of the medication from the market. A word of caution: The medical community has a dismal track record regarding medications and obesity. The disease manager's role in this is to ensure that the patient has an awareness of the risks to this therapy and closely monitors for adverse reactions.

The general consensus is that when an obese person has tried lifestyle modifications for at least 6 months, but has been unsuccessful, pharmacologic therapies may be considered. The current approved medications are listed in Table 20.5.

WEIGHT LOSS SURGERY

Gastric bypass surgery is gaining favor for the severely obese who have been unsuccessful with lifestyle management or have medical conditions that are worsened by the obesity. This surgery is known as bariatric surgery and has two primary methods: malabsorbtive and restrictive.

Table 20.5   Weight Loss Drugs Approved for Long-Term Use by the Food and Drug Administration

Drug	Dose	Mode of action	Adverse effects	Suggestions for deciding which obese patients are appropriate for the drug
Orlistat	120 mg 3×/d before meals	Inhibits pancreatic lipase to decrease fat absorption	Gastrointestinal symptoms Decreased absorption of fat soluble vitamins	Associated hypertension Associated hypercholesterolemia Difficulty removing high-fat foods from diet Frequent habit of eating at restaurants
Sibutramine	Start with 10 mg 1×/d; increase or decrease by 5 mg as needed	Norepinephrine, serotonin, and dopamine reuptake inhibitor	Can increase heart rate and blood pressure Dry mouth Insomnia Constipation Headache	History of binge eating Complaints of frequent feelings of hunger Preoccupation with food

Source: Food and Drug Administration.
Obesity Medication Approval.
www.cfscan.fda.gov/ndms/uwgqa.htm/#ther3.

Restrictive procedures close off a part of the stomach to make it smaller. The patient is left with a smaller, fully functioning stomach. After the surgery, the stomach is able to hold one ounce of food. Food absorption is not affected; the effect of this surgery is to dramatically reduce the total amount of food that can be processed at one time.

Malabsorptive procedures are the most common and involve creating a bypass from the stomach to the lower portion of the small intestine. The bypass effectively eliminates the calorie-absorbing upper portions of the intestine.

The clinical outcomes of these procedures are improving with time and experience. Weight loss up to two thirds of their excess weight after 2 years is not unusual for these patients. The patient undergoes a rigorous presurgery evaluation and postsurgery rehabilitation period.

The disease manager may be put in a position of informed decision making with the severely obese patient. If this is so, the best thing to do is to refer them to the resources at the end of this chapter or seek out local resources for the person to investigate.

CHALLENGE QUESTIONS

1. Does overweight and obesity rank in the top 10 issues for disease managers? Why?
2. How effective can a disease manager be in the weight-loss area?
3. Can a disease manager who has their own issues with weight management be effective in weight-loss strategies?

Resources

OBESITY ASSOCIATIONS
American Obesity Association
1250 24th Street, NW
Suite 300
Washington, DC 20037
800-98-OBESE (986-2373)
202-776-7711
202-776-7712 (fax)
Web: www.obesity.org
E-mail: executive@obesity.org

North American Association for the Study of Obesity
8630 Fenton Street
Suite 918
Silver Spring, MD 20910
301-563-6526
301-563-6595 (fax)
Web: www.naaso.org

OBESITY TREATMENT
American Society for Bariatric Surgery
7328 West University Avenue
Suite F
Gainesville, FL 32607
352-331-4900
352-331-4975 (fax)
Web: www.asbs.org
E-mail: info@asbs.org

American Society of Bariatric Physicians
5453 East Evans Place
Denver, CO 80222
303-779-4833 (automated referral line)
303-770-2526 (members line)
303-779-4834 (fax)
Web: www.asbp.org
E-mail: bariatric@asbp.org

Endnotes

1. National Center for Health Statistics, www.cdc.gov/faststats/ovrwt.htm. Last reviewed December 12, 2003.

2. Center for Disease Control. Obesity Trends: 1991–2001 Prevalence of Obesity Among U.S. Adults by State. Behavior Risk Factor Surveillance System (1991–2001); Self-Reported Data. www.cdc.gov/ncedphp/dnpa/obesity/trend/prev_reg.htm.

3. Revised International Table of Glycemic Index (GI) and Glycemic Load (GL) Values (2002), http://diabetes.about.com/library/membosagi/ngilists.htm. Last modified December 10, 2003.

CHAPTER 21

Get Adequate Exercise

————— OBJECTIVES —————

1. Describe the number of persons who engage in regular exercise.
2. Provide an explanation of how to discuss exercise with a sedentary person.
3. List several special considerations given to patients with chronic disease.

OVERVIEW

Exercise, and the degree of physical fitness, is a common theme during the treatment and progression of a chronic illness. The best medications, doctors, and facilities cannot begin to substitute for the positive health impact that can be had for the physically fit person. Persons who maintain a habit of exercise are rarely as ill as those who do not, so it behooves the disease manager to pay close attention to this most critical aspect of the person's health. This chapter provides the disease manager with the basic background, assessment, and intervention information necessary to add exercise to the plan of care.

REGULAR EXERCISE

Getting adequate exercise is of paramount importance to the disease manager's patients. There is substantial evidence that points to the benefits of exercise for the well to the chronically ill.

Regular exercise reduces the risk of coronary artery disease, stroke, colon cancer, diabetes, and blood pressure. Exercise also is helpful in weight loss, joint health, depression, and overall health.

Exercise can take many forms and does not have to be strenuous to return a benefit. Specific recommendations are highly dependent on the patient's

189

health status and fitness goals. At a minimum, all patients should engage in moderate intensity exercise five or more times per week.

Chronically ill patients are representative of the general population; they don't exercise as a rule. According to data in the 2001 report of the U.S. Physical Activity Statistics, about 45 percent of persons engage in moderate activity 5 or more days per week; 38 percent engage in 10 to 20 minutes of activity; 16 percent are not active at all; and 26 percent of all persons do not engage in leisure-time activity.[1]

EXERCISE COUNSELING FOR THE DISEASE MANAGER

Exercise counseling is not easy, as evidenced by inconclusive research on the topic.[2] Unless a person is a chronic exerciser, talking about and encouraging someone else to exercise can be convicting. This becomes an issue for the sedentary disease manager, quite similar to the other basic health habits except that for some reason, exercise instruction can be quite foreign and uncomfortable. This may be because disease managers come from an orientation of pathophysiology, not work or health physiology. Nurses, pharmacists, and dieticians have little or no training in exercise prescription, training principles, flexibility, and strength training. All of these are important topics to know at some level to be effective when talking about exercise. This chapter will provide enough knowledge to begin a competency in exercise counseling.

IS IT EXERCISE OR IS IT ACTIVITY?

Exercise engenders the image of a svelte man or woman running alongside of a road in the middle of nowhere. The fact is that this person is most likely an elite athlete who represents a small portion of the total exercising population. Most people who exercise regularly walk, play tennis, swim, play golf, or hike. They may sweat a little and huff and puff on the hills when pushed, but they are still exercising.

According to the *Merriam-Webster's Dictionary*, exercise is defined as bodily exertion for the sake of developing and maintaining physical fitness.[3] Activity is meant to convey something to do: quilting, vacuuming, making the bed, and playing cards are all activities. Nurses are used to using activities of daily living (ADL) to indicate functional status of a patient who is or may be impaired in some way. To be active indicates that a person is not thinking about doing something, they are doing it.

TALKING TO A SEDENTARY PATIENT ABOUT EXERCISE

As already mentioned, regular exercise is a sensitive subject. For many, fitness seems like an impossible goal. There is not a standard method for moving a person to exercise, but there are methods that appear to work better than others.

First, open up the discussion with a sense of where they are: "Mr. Jones, do you have a time during the day when you are exercising?" This is intentionally a "yes or no" question. If you plant a "no" in their mind, they will frame the rest of the discussion in terms of a gap they should fill.

Assuming a "no" answer ask, "Have you ever been in the habit of exercising?" Generally speaking, patients who have a history of exercise are much more likely to return to exercise. However, those with a lifetime of sedentary behavior have probably not "smelled" the success of feeling fit and do not have a reference point. You are asking them to travel to a place where they have never been and perhaps have never wanted to go.

For patients who have a history of prior exercise, but have fallen off the plan, the rest of the discussion should revolve around getting them back to a prior or new plan. For patients who are new to exercise, the next few steps are crucial. Say, "Exercise is a hard habit for many to adopt." Doing this acknowledges the tough place they are in and establishes a shared understanding as if the client and the disease manager were standing shoulder to shoulder. This acknowledgment also opens up a more honest discussion for the best way to achieve a fitness goal. Listen carefully to the response. Most patients will respond in agreement that exercise is not easy, is hard to do, and so forth.

Next, assess the motivation level. "Mr. Jones, do you have a desire to become more fit?" or "Mr. Jones, what do you think about becoming more fit?" The answers to this question will set the stage for what is to come. For those who have an entirely negative or neutral response, plan on returning to the discussion at a later date. The topic is firmly embedded in the patient's mind and so can be readdressed. Some patients need to dwell on tough topics before they are ready to work through them.

If the patient answers in the affirmative, move to the specifics of the motivation. Almost any reason is valid, even if they have misplaced priorities. They may say that they want to lose weight, look, feel, or even sleep better. They may want to be able to play with their grandchildren, climb the stairs that lead to the church, or go shopping without using a cart. The reasons are endless, but use the reason as an anchor for a goal to begin exercising.

Next, set a goal to begin an exercise program, and move to the exercise prescription stage.

EXERCISE PRINCIPLES

Qualifying Patient for Exercise Type and Intensity

Recommending exercise should always be under the premise that the patient does not have impending risk for worsening their condition. In some cases, too intense exercise can cause significant morbidity or even death. The best course for a disease manager is to recommend that the patient take the proposed exercise plan to the physician for their review and approval before initiating an exercise program. There are instances where a patient will require supervised exercise testing to determine heart strain or undue respiratory distress before the physician will allow exercise.

EXERCISE AND CHRONIC DISEASE

Disease managers often encounter patients who have active disease, and each of these conditions carry their own special considerations. Take care to allow for the influence of the condition when talking about a reasonable approach to fitness.

Diabetes

Diabetics should have a resting EKG and physician approval before initiating exercise.

Insulin-requiring diabetics will most likely require insulin dose and timing changes.

Insulin-requiring diabetics should have identification, an alert bracelet, and quick-acting glucose on their person while exercising.

Ensure comfortable fitting exercise footwear.

Diabetics with moderate to severe neuropathy will have challenges with weight-bearing exercise. They will not be able to sense injury to their skin and are at increased risk for injury and infection.

It is a good idea to monitor the blood glucose pre- and postexercise for a week or two to determine the usual effect of exercise.

Over time, the diabetic will lose weight that may require oral or insulin dose changes.

Good news for diabetics: The blood glucose will often return to normal or near normal levels while exercising due a remarkable increase in insulin sensitivity.

Heart Failure

All heart failure patients should have physician approval prior to exercise.

Because of the underlying pathophysiology of heart failure, exercise tolerance is compromised, sometimes severely. Exercise should be started slowly and with small realistic goals. An initial goal of walking 150 feet without shortness of breath is a common starting place.

Coronary Artery Disease

All patients with known coronary artery disease should have physician approval prior to exercise.

Signs and symptoms of heart pain should be reviewed with the patient prior to initiating an exercise program.

Nitroglycerin should be at the ready.

Osteoarthritis

Generally, exercise is beneficial for joint pain, but can cause injury when there is severe disease.

Ask the patient to confirm the exercise type, intensity, and duration with their physician if there is a suspicion of significant joint injury.

If the patient has a hip or knee replacement, reinforce the surgeon's instructions for return to activity. There is no standard recommendation for post joint replacement due to the various replacement types.

Beta blockers prevent the heart from beating too fast. For those taking beta blockers, measuring the heart rate to indicate exercise intensity is not reliable.

Obesity

Obese patients require physician approval prior to initiating an exercise plan.

Take care to begin slowly and set small goals that are realistic and designed to demonstrate progress.

Because obesity places both an internal strain on the heart and an external strain on the joints, assume that all obese patients are doing double the intensity of the nonobese person.

Weight-bearing exercise may not be feasible at the beginning of an exercise program. Instead, recommend a stationary bicycle or swimming.

Joint health is most likely compromised in an obese person. Because of this, they should walk on flat surfaces when possible to avoid undue pressure to their joints and supporting ligament and tendon structure.

Asthma

Because aerobic exercise can worsen asthma in some cases, ensure that the patient has excellent medication adherence with long-acting bronchodilators and has a short-acting inhaler available.

Inhaler use for exercise has several considerations. Short-acting inhalers act on the airways by widening them but this same mechanism causes an increase in heart rate. This means that heart rate measurements are not a reliable measure of exercise intensity and that an asthmatic with underlying coronary artery disease is at some increased risk. If this is the case, recommend a physician evaluation and approval of an exercise program.

Asthma is often aggravated by environmental triggers, so the patient should not exercise around known triggers. This may mean indoor exercising during hay fever season, for instance.

TRAINING PRINCIPLE

The training principle is also called the overload principle. The idea behind this principle is that when a patient exercises to an adequate intensity and duration, the muscle tissue will adapt to higher levels of fitness. This is accomplished through slight injury to the muscles, known as microtears, which then repair and adapt to a stronger state. It is this process that creates mild muscle soreness after exercise. If the patient has moderate to severe muscle soreness, the exercise is too intense. Because the body requires this process to gain fitness, design a fitness program that provides for gradual increases in intensity and duration and a period of rest.

EXERCISE PRESCRIPTION

Exercise prescription is a tailored plan for exercise over time that if followed will return the desired results. The process for completing an exercise prescription is relatively straightforward. The steps listed here follow a reasonable progression:

Step 1. Determine fitness goals (all that may apply).

Increase aerobic capacity

Endurance

Flexibility

Strength

Step 2. Choose a preferred and tolerable exercise or exercises. Any exercise works as long as it is does no harm to the patient from a cardiovascular or bone/joint perspective. Please refer to the special considerations section later in the chapter for more detail.

Step 3. Agree on the intensity of the exercise.

The next step in determining intensity is calculating the target heart rate (THR). The THR is a way to gauge the expected heart rate at a given intensity level. The table demonstrates what we already know: The older you get, the easier it is to describe a given intensity level as harder than it used to be! A 24-year-old has to raise their heart rate to 137 to perceive their exercise as vigorous, but for a 50-year-old, only to 119.

Make sure that the patients understand how to take their pulse on their wrist or one side of their neck. Do not allow a person to take his or her pulse using both carotid arteries and don't ask a person with significant vascular disease to take his or her pulse in their neck. Doing this may cause an embolism from plaque breaking off. Table 21.1 provides a handy target heart rate reference.

Table 21.1   Target Heart Rates by Age and Exercise Intensity

Age	Vigorous 70%	Somewhat Hard 60%	Moderate 50%	Somewhat Light 40%
18	141	121	101	81
20	140	120	100	80
22	139	119	99	79
24	137	118	98	78
26	136	116	97	78
28	134	115	96	77
30	133	114	95	76
32	132	113	94	75
34	130	112	93	74

Table 21.1 Target Heart Rates by Age and Exercise Intensity (*continued*)

Age	Vigorous 70%	Somewhat Hard 60%	Moderate 50%	Somewhat Light 40%
36	129	110	92	74
38	127	109	91	73
40	126	108	90	72
42	125	107	89	71
44	123	106	88	70
46	122	104	87	70
48	120	103	86	69
50	119	102	85	68
52	118	101	84	67
54	116	100	83	66
56	115	98	82	66
58	113	97	81	65
60	112	96	80	64
62	111	95	79	63
64	109	94	78	62
66	108	92	77	62
68	106	91	76	61
70	105	90	75	60
72	104	89	74	59
74	102	88	73	58
76	101	86	72	58

Step 4. Determine the frequency of exercise. The frequency goal is 5 days per week. There may be those who can't or won't exercise this frequently. The benefit will be less, but there will be a benefit over the long haul.

Step 5. Determine the duration of exercise. Exercise should last for 30 minutes, not including warm up, stretching, or weight training. Exercising for longer periods should be reserved for those who are willing to build up their minutes for endurance purposes. The cardiac benefit is not that much greater after 30 minutes.[4]

Step 6. Develop a plan for the exercise session. Having a set plan for how an exercise session proceeds helps with establishing a safe and productive time. The usual components are:

Warm up—3–5 minutes

Stretching—5 minutes

Table 21.2   Duration of Various Activities to Expend 150 KiloCalories for an Average 70 kg (154 lb) Adult

Intensity	Activity	Approximate duration in minutes
Moderate	Volleyball, noncompetitive	43
Moderate	Walking, moderate pace (3 mph, 20 min/mile)	37
Moderate	Walking, brisk pace (4 mph, 15 min/mile)	32
Moderate	Table tennis	32
Moderate	Raking leaves	32
Moderate	Social dancing	29
Moderate	Lawn mowing (powered push mower)	29
Hard	Jogging (5 mph, 12 min/mile)	18
Hard	Field hockey	16
Very Hard	Running (6 mph, 10 min/mile)	13

Exercise—20–40 minutes

Cool down—3–5 minutes

Stretching—3–5 minutes

Table 21.2 and the list below are helpful for the patient to understand the duration and relative intensity of various exercises.

- Washing and waxing a car for 45–60 minutes
- Washing windows or floors for 45–60 minutes
- Playing volleyball for 45 minutes
- Playing touch football for 30–45 minutes
- Gardening for 30–45 minutes
- Wheeling self in wheelchair for 30–40 minutes
- Walking 1¾ miles in 35 minutes (20 min/mile)
- Basketball (shooting baskets) for 30 minutes
- Bicycling 5 miles in 30 minutes
- Dancing fast (social) for 30 minutes
- Pushing a stroller 1½ miles in 30 minutes
- Raking leaves for 30 minutes
- Walking 2 miles in 30 minutes (15 min/mile)
- Water aerobics for 30 minutes
- Swimming laps for 20 minutes
- Wheelchair basketball for 20 minutes
- Basketball (playing a game) for 15–20 minutes
- Bicycling 4 miles in 15 minutes
- Jumping rope for 15 minutes
- Running 1½ miles in 15 minutes (10 min/mile)
- Shoveling snow for 15 minutes
- Stair walking for 15 minutes

CHALLENGE QUESTIONS

1. Can a nonexercising disease manager effectively encourage a sedentary person to start exercising?
2. How can a disease manager know that prompting a patient with chronic illness to begin exercising is safe?

Resources

U.S. Department of Health and Human Services. *Physical Activity and Health: A Report of the Surgeon General.* Atlanta, GA: U.S. Department of Health and Human Services, Centers for Disease Control and Prevention, National Center for Chronic Disease Prevention and Health Promotion, 1996.

Endnotes

1. National Center for Chronic Disease Prevention and Health Promotion. U.S. Physical Activity Statistics, 2001 State Summary Data. U.S. Department of Health and Human Services, Centers for Disease Control and Prevention, Atlanta, GA: 2002.

2. Eden, K.B. "Does Counseling by Clinicians Improve Physical Activity? A Summary of the Evidence for the U.S. Preventive Services Task Force." *Annals of Internal Medicine* 137, no. 3 (2002):208–215.

3. Merriam-Webster online, 2004. www.m-w.com.

4. Simons-Morton, D. G., Calfas, K. J., Oldenburg, B., and Burton, N. W. "Effects of Interventions in Health-Care Settings or Physical Activity on Cardiorespiratory Fitness." *American Journal of Preventive Medicine* 15 (1998):413.

CHAPTER 22

Drink Alcohol in Moderation

─────── **OBJECTIVES** ───────

1. Define alcohol dependence.
2. List the general effects that alcohol has on body systems and on people with common chronic illness.
3. In a general fashion, describe the alcohol dependence detection approach; name a common screening assessment.
4. List several tactics a disease manager can use to facilitate treatment.

OVERVIEW

The alcohol consumption habit lives on thin ice. Alcohol has protective as well as harmful properties and the line between the two is quite thin. This chapter will cover both aspects of alcohol consumption, but mainly concentrate on the alcohol dependence side of the story. The disease manager is again placed in a position to detect and then intervene and, if necessary, help the patient to put the alcohol abuse behind them. Alcoholism is a sensitive diagnosis and carries with it a wide range of emotions, social stigma, and significant morbidity. It is a progressive primary disease that negatively affects every cell of the body. Often times alcohol use starts as a behavior reserved for social occasions, but for some, the behavior evolves into a behavioral and physical dependency that is difficult to break.

Alcohol dependence symptoms are fourfold:

1. Strong craving or urge to drink.
2. Little to no control to stop drinking.

3. Physical withdrawal symptoms such as nausea, sweating, shakiness, and anxiety after stopping drinking.
4. Tolerates more and more alcohol.

DEFINITION OF ALCOHOL USE AND ABUSE

First, an alcohol drink is defined as 12 ounces of beer, 5 ounces of wine, or 1.5 ounces (a jigger) of 90-proof liquor. Alcohol use can be described as levels of harm rather than absolute volume.

Moderate Drinking

Moderate drinking, particularly of red wine, confers some degree of health protection. Moderate drinking is defined as equal to or less than two drinks a day for men and equal to or less than one drink a day for women.

Hazardous (Heavy) Drinking

Hazardous drinkers are at risk for harming themselves and others. They consume the following:

Men—greater than 14 drinks per week or 4 to 5 drinks at one sitting.

Women—greater than 7 drinks per week or 3 drinks at one sitting.

Hazardous drinkers are frequently intoxicated. They have recently been intoxicated.

Harmful Drinking

Harmful drinking causes physical or psychologic harm and is characterized by the following:

It is obvious that alcohol is responsible for such harm.

The nature of that harm can be identified.

Alcohol consumption has persisted for at least a month or has occurred repeatedly for the past year.

Alcohol Abuse

Alcohol abuse has any combination of:

Unreliable performance at work or personal obligations.

Disregard for the context for drinking; drinks in potentially dangerous situations such as drinking while driving or operating powerful machinery that requires concentration.

Law enforcement officials have been involved with incidents directly or indirectly related to alcohol abuse.

The drinking continues despite harm done to social or personal relationships.

Alcohol Dependence

Alcohol dependence is assumed if there are three or more of the following in the past year:

Drinks more alcohol to achieve "high."

Uses alcohol to relieve alcohol-related symptoms.

Cannot control the amount of alcohol consumed.

Cannot quit drinking successfully despite multiple attempts.

Has a preoccupation with drinking and will prioritize drinking activity over other activities.

Drinking habit persists with the knowledge of physical or psychological harm to oneself or others.

ALCOHOL DEPENDENCE STATISTICS

Alcohol dependence cuts through all society from the very young to the very old, the very poor to the very rich. Consider these facts from the Center for Disease Control[1]:

There were 19,817 alcohol-induced deaths in the United States in 2001, not including motor vehicle fatalities.

There were 27,035 deaths in the United States in 2001 from chronic liver disease and cirrhosis.

Chronic liver disease and cirrhosis is the 12th leading cause of death in the United States.

Sixty-three percent of Americans ages 18 and over have consumed alcohol in the past year.

Thirty-two percent of current drinkers had five or more drinks on the same occasion at least once in the past year.

Sixty percent of men 18–24 years and 42 percent of women had five or more drinks on the same occasion.

Alcohol can be a direct or indirect killer. Fortunately, alcohol-related deaths have declined. The most recent government data reveals that since 1979, the overall rate has decreased by 10 points (Table 22.1 provides more detail). The decline in alcohol-related deaths is due to many factors including public awareness campaigns, emphasis on asking about alcohol use in primary care settings, increased seat belt use, and successful alcohol-dependence treatment strategies.

Table 22.1   Number of Deaths and Age-Adjusted Death Rates per 100,000 Population for Categories of Alcohol-Related (A-R) Mortality, United States, 1979 to 1996

Year	Total		With Explicit Mention of Alcohol		Other A-R Diseases		Other A-R Adverse Effects	
	No. of Deaths	Rate	No. of Deaths	Rate	No. of Deaths	Rate	No. of Deaths	Rate
1996	110,640	32.2	19,709	6.4	45,157	9.8	45,774	16.0
1995	111,290	33.1	20,165	6.7	44,753	9.9	46,372	16.5
1994	110,754	33.6	20,075	6.8	43,976	10.0	46,703	16.8
1993	110,063	33.8	19,495	6.7	43,671	10.1	46,897	17.1
1992	107,440	33.6	19,505	6.8	42,070	10.0	45,866	16.8
1991	108,838	34.7	19,141	6.8	41,998	10.2	47,699	17.8
1990	109,751	35.5	19,672	7.2	41,738	10.3	48,342	18.1
1989	109,398	35.8	19,731	7.3	41,680	10.5	47,986	18.1
1988	108,705	36.0	18,805	7.1	41,426	10.6	48,474	18.4
1987	105,891	35.6	17,746	6.8	40,521	10.6	47,624	18.2
1986	105,792	36.0	17,367	6.7	40,524	10.8	47,901	18.6

Table 22.1 Number of Deaths and Age-Adjusted Death Rates per 100,000 Population for Categories of Alcohol-Related (A-R) Mortality, United States, 1979 to 1996 (*continued*)

Year	Total		With Explicit Mention of Alcohol		Other A-R Diseases		Other A-R Adverse Effects	
	No. of Deaths	Rate	No. of Deaths	Rate	No. of Deaths	Rate	No. of Deaths	Rate
1985	104,236	35.9	17,680	6.9	40,456	10.9	46,099	18.0
1984	103,945	36.3	17,528	6.9	40,329	11.2	46,088	18.2
1983	103,247	36.6	17,323	7.0	40,134	11.4	45,789	18.2
1982	104,702	37.8	17,455	7.1	39,864	11.5	47,384	19.2
1981	109,918	40.5	18,553	7.7	40,743	12.0	50,622	20.7
1980	112,933	42.3	19,681	8.3	41,142	12.3	52,111	21.6
1979	110,660	42.2	18,870	8.1	40,186	12.4	51,604	21.7

Source: Stinson, F. S., Nephew, T. M., Dufour, M. C., and Grant, B. F. "State Trends in Alcohol-Related Mortality, 1979–1992.[2] *U.S. Alcohol Epidemiologic Data Reference Manual,* 1st Ed. Bethesda, MD: National Institute of Alcohol Abuse and Alcoholism, National Institutes of Health (September 1996) and Unpublished AEDS data (1993–1995).

The most common underlying causes of death are detailed in Table 22.2. With the exception of the first category where the cause of death is frank alcohol use, the others represent a fairly broad spectrum of chronic diseases and accidents (Table 22.3). The disease manager would do well to keep in mind that alcohol has damaging consequences to both chronic illness and accidents.

ALCOHOL AND MEDICATION INTERACTIONS

Chronic or acute alcohol ingestion can dramatically affect the way a medication behaves. Because of how and where alcohol is metabolized, the bioavailability of a medication will be altered. This means that alcohol can enhance or reduce the effectiveness of the drug. Table 22.4 provides a summary of how selected medication classes interact with alcohol.

**Table 22.2   Alcohol-Related Underlying Causes of Death
with Associated ICD-9 Code**

Causes of Death with Explicit Mention of Alcohol
Alcoholic psychoses (291)
Alcohol dependence syndrome (303)
Nondependent abuse of alcohol (305.0)
Alcoholic polyneuropathy (357.5)
Alcoholic cardiomyopathy (425.5)
Alcoholic gastritis (535.3)
Alcoholic fatty liver (571.0)
Acute alcoholic hepatitis (571.1)
Alcoholic cirrhosis of the liver (571.2)
Alcoholic liver damage, unspecified (571.3)
Excess blood alcohol level (790.3)
Accidental poisoning by alcohol, not elsewhere specified (E860)

Other Alcohol-Related Diseases
Pulmonary and other respiratory tuberculosis (011–012)
Malignant neoplasm of lip, oral cavity, and pharynx (140–149)
Malignant neoplasm of esophagus (150)
Malignant neoplasm of stomach (151)
Malignant neoplasm of liver and intrahepatic bile ducts (155)
Malignant neoplasm of larynx (161)
Diabetes mellitus (250)
Essential hypertension (401)
Cerebrovascular disease (430–438)
Pneumonia and influenza (480–487)
Diseases of esophagus, stomach, and duodenum (530–537)
Cirrhosis of liver without mention of alcohol (571.5)
Biliary cirrhosis (571.6)
Acute pancreatitis (577.0)
Chronic pancreatitis (577.1)

Other Alcohol-Related Injuries and Adverse Effects
Motor vehicle traffic and nontraffic accidents (E810–E825)
Pedal cycle and other road vehicle accidents (E826–E829)
Water transport accidents (E830–E838)
Air and space transport accidents (E840–845)
Accidental falls (E880–E888)
Accidents caused by fire and flames (E890–E899)
Accidental drowning and submersion (E910)
Suicide and self-inflicted injury (E950–E959)
Homicide and injury purposely inflicted by other persons (E960–E969)

**Table 22.2   Alcohol-Related Underlying Causes of Death
with Associated ICD-9 Code (*continued*)**

Other Alcohol-Related Injuries and Adverse Effects (continued)
Other injuries and adverse effects
Excessive cold (E901)
Inhalation and ingestion of food causing obstruction of respiratory tract or
suffocation (E911)
Striking against or struck accidentally by objects or persons (E917)
Caught accidentally in or between objects (E918)
Accidents caused by machinery (E919)
Accidents caused by cutting and piercing instruments or objects (E920)
Accident caused by firearm missile (E922)
Poisoning by solid or liquid substances, undetermined whether accidentally or
purposely inflicted (E980)

Source: Adapted from Schultz, J., Rice, D., and Parker, D. "Alcohol-Related Mortality and Years of
Potential Life Lost—United States, 1987." *Morbidity and Mortality Weekly Report*
39 (1990):173–178.

Table 22.3   Alcohol and Chronic Illness

Condition	Alcohol Effect
Alcoholic hepatitis and cirrhosis	Alcohol is used preferentially in the liver at the expense of other metabolism. Toxic chemicals are released causing scarring called cirrhosis.
Viral hepatitis B, C	Alcoholism leads to habits that contribute to contracting hepatitis B and C.
Malnutrition	Alcohol abusers will prefer alcohol over normal eating patterns. Part of this is lifestyle related and part is vitamin and mineral deficiency caused by the alcohol itself.
Pancreatitis	Originally thought to be associated with alcoholism, but recent data says otherwise*
Esophagitis	From violent vomiting; so called Mallory-Weiss tears

Table 22.3   Alcohol and Chronic Illness (*continued*)

Condition	Alcohol Effect
Heart disease	Benefit in moderation; leading cause of death in alcoholics due to abnormal clotting factors, increased blood pressure, stroke, arrhythmias, and cardiomyopathy
Cancer	Proposed benefit in moderation; second leading cause of death for alcoholics due to potentiating the likelihood of cervical, breast, liver, and esophageal cancers to name a few.
Pneumonia	Strong association; due to changes in ability to fight off infection
Acute respiratory distress syndrome	Much more likely in alcoholics due to their predisposition to contracting pneumonia, limited immune system, and trauma
Osteoporosis	Associated with heavy drinking; related to malabsorption of calcium caused by presence of alcohol
Sleep	Affects melatonin levels to a point that disturbs normal sleep patterns
Fertility	Affects level of circulating male and female hormone
Pregnancy	Alcohol is teratogenic in nature; low birth weight common; fetal alcohol syndrome results in mental and growth retardation
Diabetes	Benefit in small to moderate amounts; alcohol can promote hypoglycemia
Peripheral neuropathy	Seen in heavy drinkers
Muscle wasting	Seen in heavy drinkers
Wernicke-Korsakoff Syndrome	Is a Thiamin (vitamin B1) deficiency; includes unsteady gait, confusion, memory difficulties

*Sarles, H. "Alcoholic Pancreatitis." In G. P. Burns and S. Banks, eds. *Disorders of the Pancreas: Controversies in Diagnosis and Management.* New York: McGraw-Hill (1992):273.

Table 22.4   Alcohol-Medication Interactions

Anesthetics	Anesthetics are administered prior to surgery to render a patient unconscious and insensitive to pain. Chronic alcohol consumption increases the dose of propofol (Diprivan) required to induce loss of consciousness. Chronic alcohol consumption increases the risk of liver damage that may be caused by the anesthetic gases enflurane (Ethrane) and halothane (Fluothane).
Antibiotics	Antibiotics are used to treat infectious diseases. In combination with acute alcohol consumption, some antibiotics may cause nausea, vomiting, headache, and possibly convulsions; among these antibiotics are furazolidone (Furoxone), griseofulvin (Grisactin and others), metronidazole (Flagyl), and the antimalarial quinacrine (Atabrine). Isoniazid and rifampin are used together to treat tuberculosis, a disease especially problematic among the elderly and among homeless alcoholics. Acute alcohol consumption decreases the availability of isoniazid in the bloodstream, whereas chronic alcohol use decreases the availability of rifampin. In each case, the effectiveness of the medication may be reduced.
Anticoagulants	Warfarin (Coumadin) is prescribed to retard the blood's ability to clot. Acute alcohol consumption enhances warfarin's availability, increasing the patient's risk for life-threatening hemorrhages. Chronic alcohol consumption reduces warfarin's availability, lessening the patient's protection from the consequences of blood-clotting disorders.
Antidepressants	Alcoholism and depression are frequently associated, leading to a high potential for alcohol–antidepressant interactions. Alcohol increases the sedative effect of tricyclic antidepressants such as amitriptyline (Elavil and others), impairing mental skills required for driving. Acute alcohol consumption increases the availability of some tricyclics, potentially increasing their sedative effects. Chronic alcohol consumption appears to increase the availability of some tricyclics and to decrease the availability of others. The significance of these interactions is unclear. These chronic effects persist in recovering alcoholics. A chemical called tyramine, found in some beers and wine, interacts with some antidepressants, such as monoamine oxidase inhibitors, to produce a dangerous rise in blood pressure. As little as one standard drink may create a risk that this interaction will occur.

Table 22.4   Alcohol-Medication Interactions (*continued*)

Antidiabetic medications	Oral hypoglycemic drugs are prescribed to help lower blood sugar levels in patients with diabetes. Acute alcohol consumption prolongs, and chronic alcohol consumption decreases, the availability of tolbutamide (Orinase). Alcohol also interacts with some drugs of this class to produce symptoms of nausea and headache such as those described for metronidazole (see "Antibiotics").
Antihistamines	Drugs such as diphenhydramine (Benadryl and others) are available without prescription to treat allergic symptoms and insomnia. Alcohol may intensify the sedation caused by some antihistamines. These drugs may cause excessive dizziness and sedation in older persons; the effects of combining alcohol and antihistamines may therefore be especially significant in this population.
Antipsychotic medications	Drugs such as chlorpromazine (Thorazine) are used to diminish psychotic symptoms such as delusions and hallucinations. Acute alcohol consumption increases the sedative effect of these drugs, resulting in impaired coordination and potentially fatal breathing difficulties. The combination of chronic alcohol ingestion and antipsychotic drugs may result in liver damage.
Antiseizure medications	These drugs are prescribed mainly to treat epilepsy. Acute alcohol consumption increases the availability of phenytoin (Dilantin) and the risk of drug-related side effects. Chronic drinking may decrease phenytoin availability, significantly reducing the patient's protection against epileptic seizures, even during a period of abstinence.
Antiulcer medications	The commonly prescribed antiulcer medications cimetidine (Tagamet) and ranitidine (Zantac) increase the availability of a low dose of alcohol under some circumstances. The clinical significance of this finding is uncertain because other studies have questioned such interaction at higher doses of alcohol.

Table 22.4   Alcohol-Medication Interactions (*continued*)

Cardiovascular medications	This class of drugs includes a wide variety of medications prescribed to treat ailments of the heart and circulatory system. Acute alcohol consumption interacts with some of these drugs to cause dizziness or fainting upon standing up. These drugs include nitroglycerin (used to treat angina) and reserpine, methyldopa (Aldomet), hydralazine (Apresoline and others), and guanethidine (Ismelin and others, used to treat high blood pressure). Chronic alcohol consumption decreases the availability of propranolol (Inderal used to treat high blood pressure), potentially reducing its therapeutic effect.
Narcotic pain relievers	These drugs are prescribed for moderate to severe pain. They include the opiates morphine, codeine, propoxyphene (Darvon), and meperidine (Demerol). The combination of opiates and alcohol enhances the sedative effect of both substances, increasing the risk of death from overdose. A single dose of alcohol can increase the availability of propoxyphene, potentially increasing its sedative side effects.
Nonnarcotic pain relievers	Aspirin and similar nonprescription pain relievers are most commonly used by the elderly. Some of these drugs cause stomach bleeding and inhibit blood from clotting; alcohol can exacerbate these effects. Older persons who mix alcoholic beverages with large doses of aspirin to self-medicate for pain are therefore at particularly high risk for episodes of gastric bleeding. In addition, aspirin may increase the availability of alcohol, heightening the effects of a given dose of alcohol. Chronic alcohol ingestion activates enzymes that transform acetaminophen (Tylenol and others) into chemicals that can cause liver damage, even when acetaminophen is used in standard therapeutic amounts. These effects may occur with as little as 2.6 grams of acetaminophen in persons consuming widely varying amounts of alcohol.
Sedatives and hypnotics ("sleeping pills")	Benzodiazepines such as diazepam (Valium) are generally prescribed to treat anxiety and insomnia. Because of their greater safety margin, they have largely replaced the barbiturates, now used mostly in the emergency treatment of convulsions.

Table 22.4   Alcohol-Medication Interactions (*continued*)

Sedatives and hypnotics ("sleeping pills") (*continued*)	Doses of benzodiazepines that are excessively sedating may cause severe drowsiness in the presence of alcohol, increasing the risk of household and automotive accidents. This may be especially true in older people, who demonstrate an increased response to these drugs. Low doses of flurazepam (Dalmane) interact with low doses of alcohol to impair driving ability, even when alcohol is ingested the morning after taking Dalmane. Because alcoholics often suffer from anxiety and insomnia, and because many of them take morning drinks, this interaction may be dangerous.
	The benzodiazepine lorazepam (Ativan) is being increasingly used for its antianxiety and sedative effects. The combination of alcohol and lorazepam may result in depressed heart and breathing functions; therefore, lorazepam should not be administered to intoxicated patients.
	Acute alcohol consumption increases the availability of barbiturates, prolonging their sedative effect. Chronic alcohol consumption decreases barbiturate availability through enzyme activation. In addition, acute or chronic alcohol consumption enhances the sedative effect of barbiturates at their site of action in the brain, sometimes leading to coma or fatal respiratory depression.

Source: Alohol-Medication Interactions. National Institute on Alcohol Abuse and Alcoholism, No. 27, PH355, January 1995.

ASSESSING FOR ALCOHOL DEPENDENCE

Assessing for alcohol use and dependence is relatively straightforward. There are a variety of standard instruments that reliably detect likelihood of alcohol dependence. The following is a suggested course of questioning and resulting actions:

Disease manager: Mr. Jones, do you drink alcohol?
Mr. Jones: Yes, I do.

There is no harm in asking the question directly. Most people don't mind talking about it. Keep the tone of your voice steady and nonjudgmental. Don't react to outrageous answers. Doing this may shut down full disclosure in a subject that is fraught with self-denial and lies.

Disease manager: How many drinks, on average, do you have a day?

Ask about volume first and put the answer in terms of average. Doing this allows the patient to answer in a way that hides heavy drinking days and will more likely return a more honest answer.

Mr. Jones: About two per day.

At face value, this is a reasonable amount of alcohol for a male. Women should only drink one drink per day.

Disease manager: How about on special occasions—like a wedding or a party? How many drinks do you have then?

This gets to binge drinking and will lead to the control question.

Mr. Jones: I do have more then. Sometimes I get into the swing of the party and can have six to eight drinks, I guess. I always wish that I didn't do that the next morning, but once I get started, it is hard for me to realize that I am drinking so much!

On the fourth question, you strike pay dirt. This question gets to binge drinking and the degree of control. Keep your voice steady and certain. Mr. Jones is realizing that he is opening up a line of questioning that will be uncomfortable. It will be important to keep the conversation professional and empathetic.

Disease manager: Do you think to have someone drive you home after that?

A little challenge to Mr. Jones—getting to the safety issue—but this also conveys a sense of caring for his safety and well-being. Most people take this line of questioning well.

Mr. Jones: Sometimes—when they are going my way. Otherwise, I take it easy and drive as carefully as I can.

Obviously this answer is problematic. Avoid the temptation to jump on this by admonishing Mr. Jones to not drink and drive because you may lose the rapport and trust built so far. Keep this in mind for the end of the conversation.

Disease manager: Mr. Jones, if you don't mind, I have a few more questions that relate to drinking alcohol.

It never hurts to ask for permission to complete your line of questioning. If Mr. Jones declines to proceed, assume the worse, and assume the presence of alcohol dependence. Return to the line of questioning on another date, but don't forget to mention the drinking-and-driving question (refer to the reference later in this monologue).

Mr. Jones: Go ahead.
Disease manager: In the past year, have you tried to cut down on drinking?

This is the first question in the CAGE assessment: cut.[1] This is a brief, four question, nonconfrontational, and accurate way to determine alcohol dependence. The ensuing three questions complete the CAGE questioning. Notice that the instrument can be delivered in a conversation without the person realizing that they are in a diagnostic mode or testing situation. If the patient answers positively to two or more questions, there is a good chance of alcoholism. There are many other alcohol screening tests. The CAGE assessment is designed to detect alcoholism, not problem drinking, so be careful not to apply the results of this screening to other situations.

Mr. Jones: No, not really.

First question is a negative response.

Disease manager: Have you been annoyed by anyone's criticisms about your drinking?
Mr. Jones: Yes, in fact just last week, my wife was talking to me about this. She said that I shouldn't have had so much to drink at the company holiday party. I didn't think I had that much; about six beers. She said I made a fool of myself, and I didn't think so.

The first positive answer; the score so far is 1. It reveals that Mr. Jones has a problem with volume and control.

Disease manager: Do you ever feel guilty about when you drink too much?
Mr. Jones: Yes, sometimes. I wish I was in a little more control.

The second positive answer; the score so far is 2.

Disease manager:	Do you ever have a drink in the morning?
Mr. Jones:	Yes, I have done that. I remember we did that in college when we had a big hangover—it helped with the symptoms. I've tried that from time to time and it works pretty well. I still feel rotten, but not as bad.

The third positive score. The final tally is 3 positive answers and it is safe to say that based upon the CAGE assessment, Mr. Jones has an alcohol dependence problem.

ALCOHOL TREATMENT OPTIONS

Once identified, the road to treatment is not easy. Because the ultimate treatment goal is total abstinence for life, lots of alcoholics resist treatment due to denial of the problem, apathy, belief that they can beat it on their own, distrust of the health care system, or lack of confidence that alcoholism can be beat. The disease manager is often the recurring voice of reason, the neutral party, and the trusted sounding board for making the decision to move forward.

Alcoholics Anonymous is a successful example of the power of confronting the issue with others who share the same problems, but getting the alcoholic to the first meeting can be difficult. Family and friends are sources of reference for the impact of the alcoholism and as long as this is done in a spirit of love and genuine concern, can be powerful motivators to entice the patient to start the road to recovery. Employers can also play a role in convincing the patient to begin treatment.

Once the decision to begin treatment is made, the disease manager may be asked to recommend treatment alternatives. There are two major treatment choices: inpatient (residential) and outpatient. Inpatient care is generally reserved for those who are heavy drinkers, have a history of severe withdrawal symptoms, have a drug use problem as well, or have health issues that predispose the patient to close clinical oversight.

Outpatient settings include interventions that range from Alcoholics Anonymous to psychological counseling or even regular physician office visits.

Whatever the treatment setting choice, to the best of their ability, the disease manager should prepare the patient for what lies ahead. Here is a short list of prequit activities:

1. Review personal reasons why the patient wants to quit, commit them to paper, and review them often with loved ones.
2. Prepare for withdrawal symptoms from an emotional and physical standpoint.

3. Prepare a plan for symptom management if the treatment is outpatient. Encourage the patient to go to their doctor, announce their plans, and talk through the medical aspects of symptom management and special considerations given their chronic condition.

4. Have the patient tell everyone they know that they will no longer be drinking after a certain date.

5. Get their term affairs in order. Pay bills and call people who have appointments or expectations in the near future to let them know that the person may be not as available as usual for a short while.

6. If the patient is smoking too, discuss whether they want to tackle both at once. Some patients will respond well to this.

7. Set realistic expectations around quit rates, relapses, changes in relationships, and changes in health status after quitting.

8. Agree on a timeframe for checking in.

CHALLENGE QUESTIONS

1. To what degree can a disease manager detect an alcohol problem over the telephone?

2. Is the disease manager the right person to spearhead care coordination for an alcoholic?

3. What is the impact of regular check-in calls to ensure quitting activity persists?

Resources

Al-Anon Family Group Headquarters, Inc., 600 Corporate Landing Pkwy, Virginia Beach, VA 23454-5617. For meetings, call 800-344-2666 in the United States or 800-443-4525 in Canada. For literature, call 800-356-9996 in the United States or 800-714-7498 in Canada. On the Internet, www.Al-Anon-Alateen.org.

Alcoholics Anonymous World Services, Inc., Grand Central Station, PO Box 459, New York, NY 10163; 212-870-3400 or www.alcoholics-anonymous.org.

American Academy of Addiction Psychiatry, 7301 Mission Road, Suite 252, Prairie Village, KS 66208; 913-262-6161 or on the Internet, www.aaap.org.

Hazelden Foundation, PO Box 11, CO3, Center City, MN 55012-0011; 800-257-7810 or 651-257-4010 from outside the United States or on the Internet, www.hazelden.org.

National Clearinghouse of Alcohol and Drug Information, PO Box 2345, Rockville, MD 20847-2345; 800-729-6686 or www.health.org.

National Council on Alcoholism, 20 Exchange Place, Suite 2902, New York, NY 10005; 800-NCA-CALL or 212-269-7797 or on the Internet, www.ncadd.org.

National Institute on Alcohol Abuse and Alcoholism, 6000 Executive Boulevard, Willco Building, Bethesda, MD 20892-7003. On the Internet, www.niaaa.nih.gov.

National Organization on Fetal Alcohol Syndrome, 216 G Street North East, Washington, DC 20002; 202-785-4585 or on the Internet, www.nofas.org.

On the Internet

Web of Addictions, www.well.com/user/woa.
Recovery, www.recovery.org/aa.

Endnotes

1. Ewing, J. A. "Detecting Alcoholism: The CAGE Questionnaire." *Journal of the American Medical Association* 252 (1984):1905–1907.

2. Arias, E., Anderson, R., Hsiang-Ching, I. C., Murphy, S., Kochanek, K. National Vital Statistics Reports. Deaths: Final Data for 2001. Volume 52, no. 3, September 18, 2003.

CHAPTER 23

Manage Stress

Damn, this traffic jam. How I hate to be late.

James Taylor

OVERVIEW

Above-average stress is the black sheep of the disease management care plan because it is so difficult to modify when present. Stress is the sum of so many variables. Some are hard-wired into the person through learned behaviors, experiences, and possibly genetics. Even so, too much stress is too much for a person with a chronic illness to bear from a clinical perspective. Although the notion of stress reduction may seem insurmountable, there are things a disease manager can do to help their patients manage stress. This chapter will show how stress affects a person with chronic illness and go through steps to help reduce stress.

STRESS

Stress is present in every living creature. Stress is the body's response to internal or external stimuli. Infection, inflammation, or psychological factors cause internal stress. Stressful environments, such as being in an argument, cause external stress. When acutely stressed, the body reacts in a predictable way. Hormones (cortisol) and catecholamines (neurotransmitters such as epinephrine and dopamine) are released in an effort to ready the body for an anticipated event. The body reacts by:

1. Heart rate increases.
2. Blood pressure increases.
3. Pupils widen.
4. Airways expand.
5. Breathing increases.
6. Immune system components of the blood are sent into the periphery.
7. Bodily fluids are redirected. Notably, the mouth fluids dry up, making it harder to swallow.
8. Blood is directed to the heart and muscles. Because of this redirection, the skin feels cool and clammy, and the scalp feels tight.
9. Digestive activity is shut down.

Two kinds of stress exist: acute and chronic. Acute stress is event driven and immediate. Running from a burning building is a good example of acute stress. Chronic stress is long term and not linked as obviously to any one event. Poor relationships, loneliness, and financial problems all contribute to chronic stress.

Stress is not necessarily a negative thing. The effects of stress aid the body in times of emergency, or even when performance has to be high such as for a public presentation or if trying to win a prize at the carnival. Chronic or long-term stress, however, can take its toll and can result in serious consequences.

Stress differs from depression and anxiety in several ways. Depression shares many of the same bodily reactions, but has an emotional component of sadness or hopelessness. Anxiety also shares many of the same bodily stress reactions, but incorporates fear or panic as a dominant emotion.

The opposite of stress is relaxation. Relaxation or the relaxation response is a known aftereffect of a stressful event or time with the bodily functions returning to their prior state. When recovering from an acutely stressful event, the relaxation response may be somewhat exaggerated. The person may even fall asleep in an effort to fully recover. Chronically stressed persons have little to no opportunity to enjoy a relaxation response. Because of this, the body's compensatory mechanisms are reset to adapt to the new order. The results of chronic stress can be significant. If the person cannot reduce or eliminate the additional stress, this can and often does lead to depression or anxiety.

Chronic stress has serious consequences in the face of chronic disease. The stress reactions create compensatory mechanisms that are not conducive to coexisting chronic illness, and with few exceptions, often worsen the person's health status. What follows in Table 23.1 is a brief summation of how chronic stress can affect chronic illness. Knowing these effects will help the disease manager understand and intervene in an appropriate manner.

Table 23.1   Effect of Stress on Selected Conditions

Condition	Effect of Stress
Alcoholism	Reduces stress; creates dependencies; interferes with diet and sleep; reduces desire for exercise
Allergies	May manifest in certain situations, like the perception that a building causes allergic symptoms such as eczema and sinus problems
Cancer	No current evidence of association with stress; positive outlook may benefit cancer patients
Diabetes	Increases insulin resistance; other stress reactions diminish the body's reaction to the disease
Dietary habits	Unusually large caffeine consumption can place a stress on the body, resulting in long-term effect on blood pressure and damage the lumen of blood vessels
Eating disorders	Mixed evidence; stress may be more of a result of the disorder than a cause
Fertility	Weak evidence that points to reduced fertility and pregnancy loss
Hair loss, unexplained (alopecia areata)	May have role
Headaches	Strong association; may not be immediate reaction; strong dependency on how the person's body reacts to stress
Heart disease	Unsure of impact; studies have shown some impact on coronary artery constriction; increased heart attack rates; increased cholesterol levels; higher blood viscosity; rhythm disorders; reduced estrogen levels; some association with hypertension and high stress levels, but evidence is mixed; angina may also be associated

Table 23.1   Effect of Stress on Selected Conditions (*continued*)

Condition	Effect of Stress
Immune disorders	Mixed effects on autoimmune diseases; conditions may improve or worsen with stress
Infections	Due to a blunted immune response, infections are more likely; everything from the common cold to HIV/AIDS are impacted; there is speculation that persons who are in chronic stress situations contract more illness in general
Inflammatory bowel disease	May cause symptom flare ups
Irritable bowel disease	Strong association
Joint or muscle pain	May increase pain; back pain in particular has been associated with increased stress levels
Memory and concentration	Very strong association, especially in acutely stressful conditions; higher levels of circulating cortisol dampens memory; short-term concentration increases are possible
Pain management	Unknown relationship; issue is complicated by a multiplicity of causal factor such as fear and personality type
Peptic ulcers	Strongly associated on anecdotal basis
Periodontal disease	Increases the risk
Pregnancy	Higher rates for pregnancy loss; negative impact on placental blood flow
Premenstrual syndrome	Weak evidence, but strong anecdotal notion that stress worsens PMS
Sexual function	Strong association with libido, erectile dysfunction

Table 23.1   Effect of Stress on Selected Conditions (*continued*)

Condition	Effect of Stress
Skin disorders	Associated with worsening eczema, psoriasis, acne, and rosacea
Sleep disturbance	Associated with insomnia and early waking due to stressful sleep
Stroke	Emerging knowledge that high-stress people, especially those who have exaggerated stress reactions, may be more likely to have a stroke
Tobacco abuse	Reduces stress in women; may increase stress in men; seek stress relief by smoking
Weight gain	Strong association; habitual eating related to stressful events; also cortisol release during stress promotes abdominal fat
Weight loss	Certain people react to stress by not eating as much

Source: Adapted from information from the National Institute of Mental Health, 6001 Executive Boulevard, Rm 8184, MSC, 9663 Bethesda, MD 20892-9663; Phone: 301-443-4513; Web site: www.nimh.nih.gov.

STRESS ASSESSMENT

The disease manager will be in a position to suggest antistress interventions. Because most patients in a disease management program have a chronic illness, managing stress to tolerable levels will reap huge rewards. It is possible to take a nonadherent, smoking, overeating, sedentary patient to a much healthier place when the stress is alleviated.

As many stress interventions exist as there are causes of stress. The first decision is to determine if the stress is significant enough to refer to a professional such as a psychologist. As a general rule, refer a patient for professional help when:

1. There are significant or unusual symptoms that occur around stressful events.

2. Stress levels are impacting several aspects of a person's life; they are in a vicious cycle.
3. Significant stressful symptoms cannot be associated with an event.
4. If the patient requests or wonders if they need professional help.

If the patient falls into one of these categories, the next step is to decide to whom to refer them. Use these as general guidelines:

1. Physician if symptoms are affecting vital bodily functions such as severe diarrhea, headaches, or chest pain.
2. Psychologist if stress reaction does not include significant physical symptoms, but is generalized to environmental factors such as relationship or job-related causes.
3. Others such as clergy when the stress is related to "purpose of life" issues and is expected to require clarification of belief systems rather than medicine or cognitive therapies.

The state of stress assessment is immature. Although there are published stress assessments, the results are hard to validate and are inconsistent. The disease manager is left to determine stress through careful questioning and synthesis of disparate information.

Stress-related questioning usually follows a secondary cause-or-effect approach where the sum of the information is more significant than any one attribute. Here are stress-related domains that the disease manager can use:

1. Daily vigor
2. Exercise pattern
3. Satisfaction with life
4. Perceived image (weight, appearance)
5. Social support
6. Variety of activities that are restful
7. Perception of quality of life
8. Have a meaningful place in life (school or work)
9. Reliance on drugs or stimulants to manage emotions or situations
10. Presence of significant life events—positive or negative
11. Self-reliance in financial and basic needs category

The Holmes and Raye Social Readjustment Rating Scale is a tool for measuring the relationship between stress and illness (Table 23.2). When using this scale, preface the life events with, "In the last 6 months, have you had any of the following?"

Table 23.2   Holmes and Raye Social Readjustment Rating Scale

	Life Event	Value
1.	Death of spouse	100
2.	Divorce	73
3.	Marital separation	65
4.	Jail term	63
5.	Death of close family member	63
6.	Personal injury or illness	53
7.	Marriage	50
8.	Fired at work	47
9.	Marital reconciliation	45
10.	Retirement	45
11.	Change in health of family member	44
12.	Pregnancy	40
13.	Sexual difficulties	39
14.	Gain of new family member	39
15.	Business readjustment	39
16.	Change in financial state	38
17.	Death of a close friend	37
18.	Change to a different line of work	36
19.	Change in number of arguments with spouse	35
20.	Mortgage over $10,000	31

Table 23.2   Holmes and Raye Social Readjustment Rating Scale (*continued*)

	Life Event	Value
21.	Foreclosure of mortgage or loan	30
22.	Change in responsibilities at work	29
23.	Son or daughter leaving home	29
24.	Trouble with in-laws	29
25.	Outstanding personal achievement	28
26.	Spouse begin or stop work	26
27.	Begin or end school	26
28.	Change in living conditions	25
29.	Revision of personal habits	24
30.	Trouble with boss	23
31.	Change in work hours or conditions	20
32.	Change in residence	20
33.	Change in schools	20
34.	Change in recreation	19
35.	Change in church activities	19
36.	Change in social activities	18
37.	Mortgage or loan less than $10,000	17
38.	Change in sleeping habits	16
39.	Change in number of family get-togethers	15
40.	Change in eating habits	15

Table 23.2 Holmes and Raye Social Readjustment Rating Scale (*continued*)

	Life Event	Value
41.	Vacation	13
42.	Christmas	12
43.	Minor violations of the law	11

Summary Scores

Score Range	Interpretation	Susceptibility
300+	Major life change	Major illness within 1 year
250–299	Serious life change	Lowered resistance to disease
200–249	Moderate life change	Depression
150–199	Mild life change	Colds, flus, occasional depression
149–0	Very little life change	Good health

Source: Holmes, T. H., and Raye, R. H. "The Social Readjustment Rating Scale." *Journal of Psychomatic Research* 11 (1967):213–218.

APPROACH TO STRESS REDUCTION

No one single best stress reduction method exists because of the wide variety of individual personality and situation possibilities. Also, be careful not to suggest stress reduction for everyday, mild stress. If a patient uses the quote at the beginning of this chapter on their way to work every day, and there are not any other issues, then it is best to do nothing. This is stress that may even be positive.

Patients may be resistant to seeking care just for stress. The prevailing attitude is that stress is a part of life and a deeply personal reaction. Some may feel that seeking care is a sign of weakness or they just "need to straighten this one thing out" to rectify the situation. Standing up for oneself is a common trait and one that is hard to get over.

CAREGIVER STRESS

Caregiver stress is common in the disease manager's world. Caregiver stress is caused by the prolonged impact of caring for a debilitated friend or family member, and can be quite severe. Caregiving wives, low-income persons, those living alone, and those caring for a severely dependent or demanding person are particularly susceptible to significant stress. For these people, seeking care is difficult for time and conscious reasons. They have devoted themselves to the last remaining time of their loved one and feel remiss in seeking care for themselves. Anyone who has been in the position of caring for a loved one knows that they are at risk for developing or worsening a chronic illness or have generally poor health.

STRESS-REDUCTION METHODS

Nonpharmacologic methods are always the preferred stress-reduction methods. A healthy approach to life is where the biggest, highest impact interventions lay. Ensure that the following are in place:

1. Adequate sleep. Patients who are sleeping well are rested and are able to cope with daily stresses—even more significant stress—in a much better way.
2. Healthy diet. A well-rounded diet creates the right balance of vitamins and nutrients to maintain optimal health. There is beginning evidence that vitamin C has a positive impact on stress levels.
3. Adequate exercise. A regular exercise plan is beneficial because it provides a respite from the daily grind and promotes relaxation. Exercise, in combination with a health diet and proper sleep, is the triad necessary for healthy living and healthy stress management.

Psychotherapy

For persons who fit the criteria for psychological intervention, a cognitive-behavioral technique can be effective. This method employs rooting out the sources of stress, a reexamination and reordering of priorities, and adopting healthier responses to stress. The process is psychologist led. It requires multiple sessions to work through the issues and to develop and maintain new behaviors.

Relaxation Techniques

Because relaxation is the enemy of the stressed, it seems good to be relaxed. Like stress, one can be too relaxed, but this usually is not a problem.

Table 23.3   Relaxation Methods

Method	Description
Meditation	A method to put the patient in an attitude of deep rest, not sleep. During meditation, breathing is slowed, and the person is relaxed as much as possible. Yoga and transcendental meditation are the most common methods.
Deep breathing	Used primarily for relaxing during times of stress rather than as a preventive measure. The classic application of this method is during childbirth. Deep breathing is an effective method, as long as the patient understands that too much deep breathing may cause hyperventilation-related problems.
Muscle relaxation	The patient alternatively tightens, then relaxes, large muscle groups one at a time. This is a good method to use to learn the feeling of being relaxed and to use when relaxation is necessary.
Biofeedback	Used to train the body to relax by controlling autonomic functions such as heart rate and breathing. Electric leads connect the patient to a monitor while the patient observes the physiologic parameters and attempts to control their functions through defined methods. The premise is that once trained, the patient is able to control stress through this learned method.

Source: Adapted from information from the National Institute of Mental Health, 6001 Executive Boulevard, Rm 8184, MSC, 9663 Bethesda, MD 20892-9663; Phone: 301-443-4513; Web site: www.nimh.nih.gov.

There are many relaxation methods; it is entirely up to the patient to determine the method that feels right and returns the most benefit.

Relaxation methods include meditation, deep breathing, muscle relaxation, and biofeedback. All of these methods promote a sense of well-being that in turn promotes relaxation. Often the patient will have to learn the technique and learn to be relaxed. It is also important to reinforce that these methods do not cure conditions associated with stress, they just reduce the impact of stress. Table 23.3 contains a short description of each technique.

MEDICATIONS FOR STRESS

No specific prescription medications for stress are available, but the disease manager may run across a patient who has been given anxiolytics agents such as Xanax and Valium or antidepressants like Elavil or Paxil as a way to manage symptoms. Encourage the patient to maintain an active discussion with their physician about the effectiveness of the medication and strive to wean them off as soon as possible. Also encourage the patient to approach their diet, exercise, and sleep patterns with zeal.

ALTERNATIVE MEDICATIONS

A plethora of herbal remedies are available to reduce stress; however, many of them are unregulated, unproven, and have a strong placebo effect. The disease manager should strongly advise the patient to be careful in their use of alternative medications because of their potential to do serious harm. Counsel the patient to monitor closely for the emergence of new signs (rash, drainage, increased urination, or constipation) or symptoms (pain or mood changes). If the patient develops anything new, prompt them to stop the medication immediately and seek their physician's care if the condition warrants.

The public has access to a wide variety of alternative medications on the Internet and at the local vitamin store. The following list is an example of what the patient might find when they visit one of the online alternative medication sites and select "Stress."

5-Htp

B Complex 100

B Complex 100 Time Release

Be-Calm

Brewer's Yeast

Calcium Citrate

Chelated Minerals

Chlorella

Hair Vitamins

Herbal Laxative

Kava Kava 300 Mg

Multiminerals Formula

No Flush Niacin

Omega 3-6-9 Efa

Potassium

Siberian Ginseng

Stress Formula

Super Multivitamin-Iron Free

Valerian

Vitamin B6

Some medications, such as 5-Htp, have been studied and have demonstrated efficacy in some studies for headaches, not stress.[1] 5-Htp also has been shown to conflict with serotonin release uptake inhibitors in a way that may cause serotonin syndrome[2] or scleroderma.[3] The bottom line is that alternative medications for stress—or any other reason—are not innocent and should be treated like any other medication.

CHALLENGE QUESTIONS

1. What is the best way to detect that a person is stressed when the interaction is by phone only?
2. Should a disease manager teach stress reduction?
3. What is the impact of stress on the elderly?

Resources

American Institute for Cognitive Therapy, 136 East 57th Street, Suite 1101, New York City, NY 10022; 212-308-2440 or www.cognitivetherapynyc.com.

The American Psychiatric Association, 1400 K Street NW, Washington, DC 20005; 888-357-7924, fax 202-682-6850, or www.psych.org.

The American Psychiatric Nurses Association, Colonial Place Three, 2107 Wilson Blvd., Suite 300-A, Arlington, VA 22201; 703-243-2443 or www.apna.org.

The American Psychological Association, 750 First Street NE, Suite 700, Washington, DC 20002-4242; www.dotcomsense.com.

The American Psychological Society, 1010 Vermont Avenue, NW, Suite 1100, Washington, DC 20005-4907; 202-783-2077 or www.psychologicalscience.org.

Association for the Advancement of Behavior Therapy, 305 Seventh Avenue, 16th Floor, New York, NY 10001-6008; 212-647-1890 or 800-685-AABT, or www.aabt.org.

National Alliance for the Mentally Ill, Colonial Place Three 2107 Wilson Blvd., Suite 300, Arlington, VA 22201-3042; 1-800-950-NAMI (6264), front desk 703-524-7600, fax 703-524-9094 or www.nami.org.

National Institute of Mental Health, 6001 Executive Boulevard, Rm. 8184, MSC 9663, Bethesda, MD 20892-9663; 301-443-4513 or www.nimh.nih.gov.

National Mental Health Association, 1021 Prince St., Alexandria, VA 22314-2971; 703-684-7722, fax 703-684-5968, or www.nmha.org.

MEDITATION SITES

Transcendental Meditation: 888-LEARN TM (532-7686) or www.tm.org.

Endnotes

1. Bolar Pharmaceutical Company. *Technical Information. L-5-hydroxytryptophan.* Corona, CA, 1984.

2. Mills, K. C. "Serotonin Syndrome." *American Family Physician* 52 (1995):1475–1482.

3. Auffranc, J. C., Berbis, P., Fabre, J. F., et al. "Sclerodermiform and Polkilodermal Syndrome Observed During Treatment with Carbidopa and 5-Hydroxytyptophan" (translated from French). *Annals of Dermatol Verereol* 112 (1985):691–692.

Avoid Tobacco

OVERVIEW

Tobacco cessation is one of the most difficult aspects of a disease manager's role. While it is true that almost every person on the planet recognizes that tobacco in any form is harmful, even fatal, a large group of tobacco users are unable or unwilling to quit. The reasons for this are complex, and it is in the disease manager's interest to have baseline knowledge and skills to understand the issues, then guide the tobacco user to become a non-user.

Tobacco cessation is not a major contributor to the disease management value proposition. This is because disease management programs are designed to produce clinical and financial impact from year to year and, in many cases, the clinical benefits are not realized for many years. There are times, of course where this is not true. Persons who have chronic obstructive pulmonary disease, asthma, or angina benefit in real time from avoiding tobacco.

This chapter will highlight the impact of smoking on one's health, describe quit methods, and provide the disease manager with aids when guiding a person through the quit process.

233

SMOKING FACTS

Based on a 2002 report from the Centers of Disease Control and Prevention, 22.8 percent, or 46.5 million, of Americans smoke cigarettes. Smoking is a habit of 18- to 44-year-olds; older persons tend to smoke less. Persons between 65 and 74 years old represent only 15 percent of all users and only 8 percent of persons over 75 still smoke.[1] There are many studies that examine smoking habits from age, race, economic, and geographic perspectives. They point to what we suspect through casual observation—the underserved, lower educated, and younger people smoke at a higher rate.

The impact of smoking is also well documented and will not be repeated here at length. Here are a few short examples. About 155,000 people died from lung cancer in 2002—this equates to about 15 percent of all people who smoke. There probably is not a person on the planet who does not realize that smoking is hazardous to their health. Disease managers are confronted with this reality every day in their patient encounters and struggle with getting the message across to the chronically ill. One of the mysteries of health counseling is paradoxical behavior such as smoking despite knowing that it is harmful.

Smoking is a direct cause of over 60,000 heart attacks per year. Smoking reduces HDL levels; causes blood vessels to become stiff; increases the tone of the blood vessels through the amphetamine in the smoke, alters essential hormone levels (women only); reduces oxygen carrying capacity; and increases the likelihood of embolism.

It is this paradox that significantly weakens most communications regarding smoking cessation. A multiplicity of factors lay between the habit and the knowledge. The dominant factor is addiction to nicotine that controls the smoker in a way that is powerful and difficult from which to break free. In this and many other cases, knowing does not lead to behavior. Table 24.1 provides a brief summary of how smoking affects common conditions encountered by a disease manager.

LIKELIHOOD OF QUITTING SMOKING

Fortunately, it is possible to stop smoking. Because the smoking issue is one of many that the disease manager will tackle, it is helpful to know the odds of quitting based on patient attributes.

Patients who will have the toughest time quitting include heavy smokers, those who inhale deeply, have a long smoking history, have had severe withdrawal reactions with prior quitting experiences, are female, and/or have a tendency to cheat when quitting.[2]

Table 24.1   Effects of Smoking on Selected Conditions

Condition	Effect of Smoking
Alzheimer's Disease	Might have protective effects, but the evidence is mixed
Baldness	Associated with some forms of balding
Bladder Cancer	Higher rates in women smokers
Breast Cancer	No current evidence of causation, but may worsen existing cancer because of tendency to metastasize to the lung
Bronchitis and Emphysema (COPD)	Strongly associated with this and almost any chronic lung disease
Cancer	Obviously linked to many cancers. About 85 percent of all lung cancers directly linked to smoking; a relatively low survival rate once found. Women more likely to contract lung cancer than men; female smokers have more lung cancer than breast cancer.
Cataracts	Increased likelihood of cataract surgery in smokers
Cervical Cancer	About a third of cervical cancers have been linked to a smoking habit
Colon Cancer	Linked to long-term smokers
Crohn's Disease	Higher rates in smokers
Diabetes	Combination of type 2 diabetes and a smoking habit dramatically accelerates heart vessel damage and also reduces kidney function; diabetes complications such as neuropathy, nephropathy, and blindness all hastened by smoking
Diverticulitis	Mostly a condition of people over 50 years old; smoking strongly associated with this condition that has serious bleeding and infection complications

Table 24.1   Effects of Smoking on Selected Conditions (*continued*)

Condition	Effect of Smoking
Environmental exposure to smoke	Smoke is the most caustic part of the cigarette; persons exposed to environment tobacco smoke at increased risk for many conditions mentioned here
Esophageal and Mouth Cancer	Smokers have higher rates
Gum Disease	Peridontitis, or infection of the gums, more prevalent in smokers than nonsmokers
Hearing Loss	Due to a reduced blood flow in the middle ear, high frequency hearing loss most common
Heart Disease and Stroke	Smokers at significantly higher risk for heart disease or stroke; even light smokers (3–6 cigarettes per day) double their risk; women at more risk than men, especially those taking oral contraceptives
Hepatitis	Associated with smoking, excessive drinking that results in liver scarring known as cirrhosis
Hyper/Hypothyroidism	Strongly associated with increased rates of these conditions
Incontinence	Women who smoke twice as likely to develop urinary incontinence
Kidney Cancer	Higher rates in smokers
Low Back Pain	A higher incidence of chronic low back pain
Oral Cancer	Higher rates in smokeless and cigarette smokers
Osteoporosis	Smoking interferes with the formation of new bone, so female smokers at a higher risk for osteoporosis; older women who smoke often have higher risk of hip fracture
Pancreas Cancer	Higher rates in smokers

Table 24.1   Effects of Smoking on Selected Conditions (*continued*)

Condition	Effect of Smoking
Parkinson's Disease	Lower incidence in smoking cessation; thought to be related to some form of protection conferred by the nicotine
Peptic Ulcers	Studies show both an aggravating and neutral effect with smokers
Skin Cancer	Smokers at triple the risk
Stomach Cancer	Higher rates in smokers
Ulcerative Colitis	Lower rates in smokers
Wound healing, surgery recovery	Because smoking limits oxygen-carrying capacity and impairs other healing factors, recovery lengthened (If a smoker quits about 2 months prior to surgery, their wound healing improves dramatically)
Wrinkles	Smokers, especially in certain ethnic groups, develop more severe wrinkles

WOMEN AND SMOKING

Women have a tougher time than men when it comes to quitting smoking. This is regretful considering the higher lethality of tobacco use in women. The reasons it is harder for them to quit are complex but speculation is that women do not respond as well to nicotine patches as men, fear the possible weight gain more, cannot use nicotine patches while pregnant, undergo hormonal changes that alter the effectiveness of nicotine replacement aids, and often fear a loss of control that smoking confers.[2]

SMOKING CESSATION AND WEIGHT GAIN

It is true that smokers are likely to gain more weight than they anticipated when they quit. Some of the reasons for this are metabolic in nature, and some are a result of coping with withdrawal symptoms. When a patient quits smoking, they lose the metabolic impact of nicotine, which is approximately 200 calories per day. If the patient does not change their eating or exercise habits, this results in gaining one pound every 17½ days. Add to this the tendency to snack more, the metabolic changes in insulin levels, and a lower basal metabolic rate, and the rate of weight gain likely will be higher.

Increasing the exercise level when quitting is the best recipe for minimal weight gain. Even a 15-minute walk along with more careful eating will make a huge difference in the outcome. There is also evidence that during the time in use, nicotine replacements protect against weight gain. This makes sense given the effects of nicotine on the body.

NICOTINE IS ADDICTIVE

Nicotine is extremely addictive. Interestingly, nicotine acts similarly to heroin and cocaine. There are some who feel that nicotine has the same addictive power as heroin.[3] Nicotine can act as a stimulant or depressant. It can create a sense of well-being, may enhance memory, and has antidepressant qualities. All of these effects are temporary—lasting for as long as the nicotine is circulating in the bloodstream and at the correct levels. Long-term smokers report that they smoke more intensely as the day progresses. Researchers believe this is because the body becomes desensitized to the effects of nicotine as the day wears on, necessitating the need for more of the drug.

WITHDRAWAL SYMPTOMS

One of the things disease managers hear all the time from smokers who are trying to quit is that they have never felt worse than when they try to quit. The emergence of withdrawal symptoms creates confusion and discouragement, which in turn leads to relapses to relieve the symptoms. Because nicotine is an extremely potent psychoactive drug, withdrawal symptoms can emerge within hours of quitting. Most smokers report that the symptoms are the most intense for the first 3 to 5 days, then disappear after 2 to 3 weeks.[4] There are some who report waves of symptoms for years after quitting.

The usual withdrawal symptoms are headaches, coughing, indigestion, sweating, tingling in the hands or feet, emotional outbursts, confusion, irritability, anxiousness, disrupted sleep, and depression.[4] Not all smokers will have all these symptoms, but it is not unusual for them to have many of them—especially long-term smokers. Disease managers would be wise to point this out to patients who are about to quit so they can prepare mentally for a rather rough road ahead. Disease managers should be particularly aware of the degree and time frame of depressive symptoms. For some smokers, the depression mimics mourning and is temporary; others develop full-blown major depression that may require therapy to reverse.

APPROACHES TO SMOKING CESSATION

Having a good knowledge of smoking cessation strategies is important for the disease manager. Because this process can be very easy or very hard, knowing which road the patient will be on will help determine if the quitting process is best handled by the disease manager or by another resource. The following line of questioning will help to decide on a course of action:

Disease manager: Mr. Jones, do you have a desire to quit smoking?

Mr. Jones: Yes, I do, but I don't know how I'm going to do it.

If a patient indicates a desire, then ask about past experiences. If they do not want to quit, plant the seed that you are willing and able to help him when he does. It make take many conversations before the patient makes the decision. If the patient senses that you are disappointed in a "not at this time" response, then they may question your desire to help them. Be careful to be empathetic and nonjudgmental.

Disease manager: There are several successful methods for quitting smoking. What have you tried in the past?

Mr. Jones: I have tried on my own to quit—cold turkey—but I couldn't get past the second day because I got terrible headaches and my heart started to pound. My wife tells me that I looked like I was having a heart attack!

Mr. Jones is telling you that he has tried before and has had significant symptoms. Unfortunately, this does not bode well for Mr. Jones; patients who have problems with withdrawal are less likely to be successful at quitting. The fact that his heart is pounding may indicate he has a cardiovascular sensitivity to nicotine.

Disease manager: Have you picked a method and a quit date?

Mr. Jones: I don't know about the quit date, but I'm wondering about the patches.

This conversation is going well. Choosing a method and quit date are extremely important. Patients who don't have a plan are not likely to quit successfully. This is a chance to discuss smoking cessation methods, and Mr. Jones is leaning toward one of the most successful ones.

Disease manager: Let's go through your options for persons who are trying to quit smoking. . . .

Patients who quit *cold turkey* (suddenly) have a relatively dismal quit rate. On average, this works for only 4 percent of patients.[4] If the patient is resolute that this will be their method, prepare them for symptom management. Also recommend that they purchase educational and behavioral material that will help them to work through the many issues they are about to face.

Patients who ask for nicotine replacement are choosing one of the more successful methods. Nicotine supplements are designed to deliver a set amount of nicotine to the bloodstream without the usual other contaminants. Nicotine supplementation is most effective for smokers who are moderate to heavy users. If a person smokes less than 15 cigarettes per day, this method is not useful. Also, the best chance of success using nicotine replacement is to combine it with an established monitoring program that provides ongoing support.

At present, 75 percent of health plans do not reimburse for nicotine replacement, so most patients will purchase them at retail outlets.[5] Nicotine replacement is available in slow-release patches, gum, inhalers, and nasal sprays. Each of these products comes with quitting tips, a list of adverse effects, and full-use instructions. If smoking cessation is a common discussion, then it would behoove the disease manager to have the inserts from a variety of products they typically recommend. Nicotine replacement is safe for most people with heart disease or diabetes and adolescents. Nicotine replacement is not safe during pregnancy. No one should use this method over the long term.

Medications Related to Smoking Cessation

Bupropion (Zyban), a prescribed medication, is the primary medication used for smoking cessation. It acts by increasing the effects of dopamine, a neurotransmitter that is associated with nicotine addiction. The usual dose is 150mg twice a day given over 7 to 12 weeks. The quit rates for Zyban vary based on the presence of other aids, such as nicotine replacement patches and counseling support. Generally speaking, there is a 20 to 25 percent quit rate with Zyban, and up to 35 percent with enhanced support systems.[6] Patients will also tend to maintain their weight better while on the drug. With patients who are not depressed, Zyban will lift their mood even further, creating a feeling of more energy and a pleasing demeanor.[6]

Other medications given as quitting aids are considered investigative. They are Clonidine, Nortriptyline, and Naltrexone and are showing some promising results.[4] For the most part, these medications act on the central nervous system to mitigate the urge to smoke and reduce the impact of depression. Like any central nervous system depressants, they have a sedative effect.

STRATEGIES FOR SMOKING CESSATION

1. Choose a method that allows a patient to stop smoking on a certain date. Patients who choose to reduce the number of cigarettes slowly over time have a much harder time quitting.

2. Have the patient write down a list of reasons to quit smoking and have them place this list in a public place to refer to every day. This can take the form of a contract. Some patients need to do this; some don't.

3. Provide anticipatory guidance to help the patient work through the upcoming withdrawal symptoms. Suggest that they:

    a. Tell as many people as possible that they have quit.

    b. Have a strategy to beat the cravings.

    c. Use nicotine replacement medication as prescribed.

    d. Plan for increased exercise. Relaxation with stretching is a good antidote for reducing anxiety.

    e. Plan for a healthy diet to include plenty of water and healthy snack foods.

    f. Identify, and then eliminate, routines that contribute to habitual cigarettes. This may mean not taking breaks with friends who smoke during the sensitive withdrawal period or staying away from smoky environments such as bars and bowling alleys.

    g. Maintain full communication with their physician.

CHALLENGE QUESTIONS

1. When should a disease manager refer a patient to a smoking cessation program?

2. How much time should a disease manager devote to smoking cessation counseling sessions?

3. Given the relatively short time frame in the value proposition for disease management, what value does smoking cessation bring?

Resources

Agency for Health Care Research and Quality, Publications Clearinghouse, 2101 E. Jefferson St., Suite 501, Rockville, MD 20852; 301-594-1364 or www.ahcpr.gov.

American Academy of Addiction Psychiatry, 7301 Mission Road, Suite 252, Prairie Village, KS 66208; 913-262-6161 or www.aaap.org.

American Academy of Medical Acupuncture, 4929 Wilshire Boulevard, Suite 428, Los Angeles, CA 90010; 323-937-5514 or www.medicalacupuncture.org. To find an acupuncturist, go to www.medicalacupuncture.org/refsearch.html.

American Cancer Society, 1599 Clifton Road, NE, Atlanta, GA 30329; 800-ACS-2345, 404-320-3333, or www.cancer.org.

The American Council on Science and Health, 1995 Broadway, Second Floor, New York, NY 10023-5860; 212-362-7044 or www.acsh.org. Offers useful information on the health consequences of smoking.

The American Lung Association, 1740 Broadway, New York, NY 10019-4374; 800-LUNG-USA (212-315-8700) or www.lungusa.org.

The American Society of Clinical Hypnosis, 130 East Elm Court, Suite 201, Roselle, IL 60172-2000; 630-980-4740 or www.asch.net. To find a reliable hypnotherapist, send a self-addressed stamped envelope to the society.

National Cancer Institute, 6116 Executive Boulevard, Suite 3036A, MSC8322, Bethesda, MD 20892-8322; 800-422-6237 or www.nci.nih.gov. The NCI offers free information on how to quit smoking.

Nicotine Anonymous World Services; 866-536-4539 or www.nicotine-anonymous.org. The organization uses the same principles as Alcoholics Anonymous, and it offers a directory of meeting places and times in many locations.

The Society for Clinical and Experimental Hypnosis, 3905 Vincennes Rd., Suite 304, Indianapolis, IN 46268; sunsite.utk.edu/IJCEH/scehmain.htm.

Web Sites

No Smoke Home Page: www.smokefreekids.com/smoke.htm.

Philip Morris USA: www.pmusa.com/health_issues/quitting_smoking.asp.

QuitNet: www.quitnet.com/qn_main.jtml.

Endnotes

1. Centers for Disease Control and Prevention (CDC). Annual Smoking-Attributable Mortality, Years of Potential Life Lost, and Economic Costs—United States, 1995–1999. *MMWR Morb Mort Wkly Rep.* 51 (2002):300–303. Available online at www.cdc.gov/mmwr//preview/mmwrhtml/mm5114a2.htm. Accessed October 2003.

2. Office of the US Surgeon General. Reducing Tobacco Use: A Report of the Surgeon General. Centers for Disease Control and Prevention (CDC), Office on Smoking and Health. 2000. Available online at www.cdc.gov/tobacco/sgr/sgr_2000/index.htm. Accessed October 2003.

3. Centers for Disease Control and Prevention (CDC), National Center for Chronic Disease Prevention and Health Promotion. Toxic Chemicals in Tobacco Products. Available online at www.cdc.gov/tobacco/research_data/product/objective21-20.htm. Accessed October 2003.

4. U.S. Department of Health and Human Services. Reducing Tobacco Use: A Report of the Surgeon General. Centers for Disease Control and Prevention (CDC), Office on Smoking and Health. 2000. Available online at www.cdc.gov/tobacco/sgr/sgr_2000/index.htm. Accessed November, 2003.

5. Fiore, M. C., Smith, S. S., Jorenby, D. E., Baker, T. B. The effectiveness of the nicotine patch for smoking cessation. A meta-analysis. *Journal of the American Medical Association.* 273, no. 3 (1995): 181.

6. Hurt, R. D., Sachs, D. P. L., Glover, E. D. et al. A comparison of sustained-release bupropion and placebo for smoking cessation. *New England Journal of Medicine,* 337 (1997): 17.

Prevent Accidents

OVERVIEW

Because disease managers work primarily with chronically ill persons who have ever-evolving physical and mental limitations, accident prevention becomes important. Almost all accidents result in either an injury or perhaps death. The disease manager is in a position to recognize and anticipate certain accident risks and make recommendations to ameliorate those risks. Because the value proposition for disease management depends on the degree to which the person remains healthy, ignoring accident prevention can undermine all other interventions that focus on self-care and best practices. This chapter explores a range of physical and psychological limitations and processes that are associated with chronic illness or the aging process and provides strategies to prevent accidents that are likely to occur as a result of those limitations. Because of their prevalence and relative importance to disease management practice, medication errors are another form of unintentional injury and are focused on at the end of this chapter.

243

ACCIDENT FACTS

Accidents can cause significant morbidity and mortality. In fact, when considered against the top 10 causes of all deaths, as shown in Table 25.1, unintentional injury ranks fifth on the list, ahead of diabetes, the most prevalent disease management program.

According to a recent study, approximately 11 percent of all outpatient visits were as a result of an injury, the fourth most common reason to make an outpatient visit behind chronic conditions, acute conditions, and preventive health[1]. Emergency departments are, of course, the primary locations for injury care. Refer to Table 25.2 for a list of the types of injuries (their frequency in parentheses) seen in the emergency room. This data does not reflect the innumerable close calls and nontreated injuries that persons incur.

Table 25.1   The Top 10 Leading Causes of Death, United States 2002, All Races, Both Sexes (All Ages) (incidence per year in parentheses)

1. Heart Disease (700,142)
2. Malignant Neoplasms (553,768)
3. Cerebro-vascular (163,538)
4. Chronic Low Respiratory Disease (123,013)
5. Unintentional Injury (101,537)
6. Diabetes Mellitus (71,372)
7. Influenza and Pneumonia (62,034)
8. Alzheimer's Disease (53,852)
9. Nephritis (39,480)
10. Septicemia (32,238)

Source: Center for Disease Control. *10 Leading Causes of Nonfatal Injury, United States 2002, All Races, Both Sexes, Disposition: All Cases,* Office of Statistics and Programming, National Center for Injury Prevention and Control, CDC National Center for Health Statistics Vital Statistics System 2002, www.cdc.gov/ncipc/wisqars/nonfatal/quickpicks/quickpicks_2002/allinj.htm. Accessed April 2004.

Table 25.2   Unintentional Injuries for 2002 in the United States

Total Unintentional Injuries (26,622)
Falls (7,034)
Struck against or struck accidentally by objects or persons (4,513)
Motor vehicle, traffic (4,216)
Cutting or piercing by instruments or objects (2,518)
Overexertion and strenuous movements (1,521)
Natural and environmental factors (1,505)
Poisoning by drugs, medicinal substances, biological, or other solid and liquid substances, gases, and vapors (700)
Fire and flames, hot substances or objects, or caustic or corrosive material and steam (564)
Motor vehicle, nontraffic (429)
Pedal cycle, nontraffic and other (411)
Machinery (305)
Other transportation (139)

Source: McCaig, L. F., and Burt, C. W. National Hospital Ambulatory Medical Care Survey: 2002 Emergency Department Summary. *Advance Data from Vital and Health Statistics*, no. 340. Hyattsville, MD: National Center for Health Statistics, 2004.

COMMON PHYSICAL AND PSYCHOLOGICAL LIMITATIONS

One can imagine that physical and psychological limitations can place a person at a higher risk for injury. These limitations include memory loss, inability to concentrate, poor vision, hearing loss, poor balance, loss of strength, loss of flexibility, loss of the sense of smell, and loss of the sense of touch. Not everyone with a chronic illness has all of these limitations, but many have at least one of them.

Assessing for the presence of these limitations is not difficult. The disease manager only has to ask the following:

Disease manager: Mr. Jones, do you struggle with any of the following?

- Keeping important things in mind such as remembering to turn the stove off or locking your house before you go to bed?
- Concentrating on tasks that require you to work safely such as cutting vegetables or operating lawn equipment?
- Seeing clearly enough to move around, perform routine tasks, or drive?
- Hearing sounds that serve to alert you such as a doorbell, whistling tea pot, or a timer on an oven?
- Maintaining your balance while moving around or standing still?
- Having the strength to carry objects such as grocery bags?
- Having the flexibility to stoop over or bend to pick something up?
- Having enough sense of smell to detect propane gas, smoke, or chemical odors?
- Having enough sense of touch to distinguish hot or cold water or smooth or rough surfaces?

If the person responds in the affirmative to any of these, consider providing instructions and interventions to minimize the likelihood of an accident. Think back to the types of injuries listed in the prior section. Most of them can be traced to operating machinery, driving, falling, or manipulating a sharp object. In almost all cases, an accident involves an actor, an implement, and a situation. It is up to the disease manager to determine if the actor (the patient) can handle the implement (car, knife, ladder, or lawnmower) in the situation (physical or psychological limitations). The remaining sections of this chapter provide background knowledge and interventions that will be useful to the disease manager.

Memory

Forgetting important things is high on the list of accident prevention. If the person relates a pattern of forgetfulness, ensure that they have a caretaker to keep watch over their activities. The best method of prevention is to speak with that caretaker about items that may cause harm, such as toasters, ovens, stoves, irons, and power tools. If possible, ask that the person not use them at all. If this is not possible, then suggest that other arrangements be made that will eliminate the need for using the devices in question or ensuring that the appliances have safety switches or automatic turn-off features.

Concentration

Concentration demands a clear mind. Persons who have early dementia, have Parkinsonism, or are taking medications that depress the central nervous system are clearly at risk for having a lack of concentration. The person should recognize that they have a concentration problem and adjust their activities accordingly. Suggest that their actions be slow and deliberate, thinking through each step before they take it.

Vision

Poor vision can lead to many accidents. Elderly persons have limited vision, especially at night, and are prone to car accidents in low light. Diabetics with advanced retinopathy or those with macular degeneration have poor vision overall. Even simple tasks, such as cooking a meal or navigating a flight of poorly lit stairs, can be a challenge.

Suggest that those with night vision problems (almost all persons over 75 years old) not drive after dusk. Also ask that proper lighting be installed along the main traffic areas of the house, especially in the kitchen, bathroom, and around the stairs. For those with cataracts, suggest that they be evaluated for cataract removal.

Hearing

Not hearing well leads to a lack of awareness of one's surroundings. Simple auditory alerts such as kitchen timers, tea pots, or car horns blowing can prevent significant injury. The obvious intervention is to suggest a hearing and hearing aid evaluation, but this may not be enough. Suggest that, where possible in the home, visual reminders are used in addition to auditory ones. These might include timers with lights or doorbells that chime and cause a light to blink. Also suggest that persons who have severe to complete hearing loss that is not corrected not drive.

Balance

Loss of balance is a precursor to falling, and for too many elderly persons, significant morbidity and mortality. If the disease manager suspects that balance is an issue, recommend a medical evaluation as well as an intervention that includes the use of walking devices such as canes, walkers, or scooters. Suspect that the person has balance problems if they tell you that they have to hold on to another person or a wall to get around.

Muscle Strength

Muscle strength diminishes over the years, and by the time a person reaches their seventies they are relatively weak. Most persons realize this and make accommodations, but others do not. The best recommendation is to encourage the person to maintain the highest level of fitness possible so they can perform the usual activities of daily living such as shopping, light yard work, and housework. It is never too late to increase muscle strength. Persons who are weak are prone to injuring themselves by lifting too much weight or attempting to support themselves in an unusual position. Both of these situations lead to accidents caused by exhaustion of strained muscles.

Flexibility

Older persons typically lose quite a bit of flexibility in the long muscles of their legs and back. This results in rigidity that may limit the person's ability to avoid an otherwise avoidable accident. Ask the person if they are able to tie their shoes without sitting on a chair, or if they are able to stretch their leg out on an ottoman without feeling tight. Like muscle strength, flexibility can be regained with retraining. Suggest that the inflexible person do slow, steady leg and back stretches every day, cautioning them to stretch in a safe position such as sitting on a chair or on the floor.

Sense of Smell

Like the rest of the senses, the sense of smell diminishes with age. In some, it becomes quite blunt and only the strongest odors are detected. This is unfortunate because accidents such as gas leaks and fires are quite often smelled before they are seen. The fortunate solution for this limitation is to ensure that fire, carbon monoxide, and gas sensors are installed in the right places and that they are working.

Sense of Touch

The ability to determine that an object is hot or cold, smooth or rough, or to feel the object at all is critical to avoiding unnecessary injury. The sense of touch is primarily an issue for those with diabetic neuropathy, but there are many other reasons why a person can have a diminished sense of touch. Most often, the person is well aware that they cannot feel things as well as they should and will be careful around potentially harmful situations. The primary caution is to be aware of hot bath water and unnoticed skin friction caused by ill-fitting shoes or clothes. Water temperature gauges are available to monitor bath water. Also, the person can reduce the temperature of the water heater to prevent excessively hot water.

The Disease Manager's Role

The primary skills for the disease manager in accident prevention are anticipation and intervention. Although most disease managers do not consider accident prevention as a significant part of their practice, it deserves attention when the situation warrants.

MEDICATION ERRORS

The disease manager is often in a position to detect medication errors. In a sense, a medication error is an accident that is avoidable. Medication errors are one of the nation's leading causes of morbidity and mortality, accounting for as many as 98,000 deaths per year in hospitalized patients alone.[2] Because the typical disease management patient takes multiple medications, a mechanism to detect and act on potential medication errors is an important part of the approach.

Here are some helpful strategies to prevent medication errors:

1. Ensure that the patient has a master list of all medications that includes the patient's name, dosage, directions, prescribing physician's name, and reason for taking that has been reviewed and confirmed by their primary care physician. Make sure that the list includes nonprescription medications and anything else that the patient takes or applies to affect their health. The master list should also include all known drug allergies or sensitivities. Also, remind the patient that this master list should be reviewed at regular intervals. This is by far the most effective step a disease manager can take to prevent medication errors.

2. Encourage the patient to do the following when they are handed a prescription:
   a. Ensure that the physician has reviewed the master list prior to prescribing the medication.
   b. Listen carefully to the physician when they are talking about the medication.

    c. Try to read the prescription. If the patient cannot read it, then chances are the pharmacist will have trouble reading it.

    d. Ask about the purpose of the medication, how to take it, side effects to watch for, potential interactions with current medications, and any diet or activity limitations.

    e. Ask about what to do if there is a problem with the medication.

    f. If there is a history of misunderstanding, a problem with comprehension, or the patient is hard of hearing; it will be best to have someone else present to listen as well.

    g. Clarify that the medication is for a certain time period or will be taken on a chronic basis. Many patients stop taking medications because they mistakenly think that the condition is cured. Stopping cholesterol lowering medications once cholesterol levels have returned to normal levels is an instance particularly prone to this phenomenon.

3. Re-ask the pharmacist the same questions about the details of the medication(s). Ensure that the medication is in fact filled exactly as the physician ordered. This step is extremely important because a large percentage of medication errors involve misinterpreting the original prescription.

4. Ask about what happens if the medication needs to be stopped suddenly. There are some medications that should be tapered off or they may cause severe symptoms if stopped too abruptly.

5. Do not leave the pharmacy before there is a clear understanding of how to take the medication. Ask for a written explanation. Most pharmacies offer this service.

6. If the medication requires measuring liquid, ensure that the correct applicator is obtained.

7. If the patient is about to have a procedure, counsel them to go to the highest volume, most experienced setting possible. There are fewer medication-related errors when the process is mature.

8. Many medication errors are a result of poor discharge planning. Quite often, the discharge plan contains new medications that are explained by a staff nurse. If there is any question about the medication, contact the prescribing physician for clarification.

9. Encourage the patient to be as open as possible about sensitive-topic side effects such as loss of erection or libido. Patients may not understand that there are options to minimize side effects.

10. In addition to the medication list, keep a basic health history with the patient at all times. This will require generating a standard form for patients to carry with them. Because there can be several versions of medical records—contributing to potential errors in judgment—a basic health history form will reduce the incidence of medication errors. See Figure 5.1 for an example of a health history form.

Figure 25.1   Example Medication List and Health History Form

Name:_____

Address:_____

Date of Birth:_____

Telephone:_____

Emergency Contact:_____

Blood Type:_____

Date last reviewed with physician:_____

Physicians

Physician Name	Contact Information	Specialty

Medical Conditions

Medical Conditions	Onset Date	Resolved

Figure 25.1   Example Medication List and Health History Form (*continued*)

Medication List

Medication Name	Dose	Instructions	Reason	Prescriber

Allergies/Sensitivities

Allergies/Sensitivities	Reaction	Onset Date

Past Surgeries or Procedures

Past Surgeries or Procedures	Date	Result

Figure 25.1 Example Medication List and Health History Form (*continued*)

Immunizations (Adult)

Immunization	Last Immunization Date
Tetanus	
Pneumoccal Vaccine	
Flu Vaccine	
Hepatitis A	
Hepatitis B	
Measles	

CHALLENGE QUESTIONS

1. Should a disease manager evaluate the accident risk for all their patients?
2. How can a telephonic disease manager objectively determine the degree of limitation—and thus know the likelihood of an accident—without a face-to-face visit?
3. What are the sources of savings for accident prevention? Are they significantly high enough to address?

Endnotes

1. Hing ES, Middleton, KR. National Hospital Ambulatory Medical Care Survey: 2001 outpatient department summary. Advance data from vital and health statistics; no 338. Hyattsville, MD: National Center for Health Statistics. 2003.
2. Subramanian S, Kellum JA: Limiting harm in the ICU. Minerva Anestesiol. 2000; 66: 324–332.

Index